Postponing Parenthood

The Effect of Age on Reproductive Potential

Postponing Parenthood

The Effect of Age on Reproductive Potential

Gale A. Sloan, R.N.

Foreword by
Paul B. Marshburn, M.D.

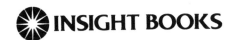 **INSIGHT BOOKS**

Plenum Press • New York and London

Library of Congress Cataloging-in-Publication Data

Sloan, Gale A.
    Postponing parenthood : the effect of age on reproductive
  potential / Gale A. Sloan ; foreword by Paul B. Marshburn.
        p.   cm.
    Includes bibliographical references and index.
    ISBN 0-306-44466-6
    1. Infertility, Female--Age factors. 2. Pregnancy in middle age.
  I. Title.
    [DNLM: 1. Aging--physiology. 2. Fertility--physiology.
  3. Parents--psychology. 4. Reproduction--physiology.   WQ 205
  S634p]
  RG201.S66   1993
  618.1'78--dc20
  DNLM/DLC
  for Library of Congress   92-48286
                                                                CIP

ISBN 0-306-44466-6

Insight Books is a division of Plenum Publishing Corporation
233 Spring Street, New York, N.Y. 10013

An Insight Book

Printed in the United States of America

To Bob

Foreword

Every day in my practice as a reproductive endocrinologist, I meet with couples who are confused and frustrated by their inability to conceive. Most are psychologically, physically, and financially capable of caring for a child; yet, they haven't been able to get pregnant. Even though we live in a time when the area of reproductive medicine is exploding with new technologies for helping couples conceive, not all couples are well served by these advances. Some couples are simply unprepared for how intensive, time-consuming, and expensive these treatments are. Others still can't conceive, despite these new treatments.

For these reasons, I feel that *Postponing Parenthood* should prove a valuable guide for couples who are considering becoming parents, whether now or some time in the future. In writing this book, Gale Sloan performed extensive research and crystallized a mountain of facts to shed light on the pros and cons of postponing parenthood. Together, we examined each page of the manuscript to ensure that you receive the most accurate and up-to-date information available. What has resulted is a book that is clear, concise, and easy to read, and which contains the information that every couple should have when making important decisions about when to become parents.

In the early chapters of the book, Gale Sloan presents interesting social and psychological aspects of parenthood at various ages. She then addresses the most pressing questions regarding aging and infertility. To what extent does age affect your ability to become pregnant? How can you preserve your reproductive function? How can you facilitate pregnancy once you start trying to conceive? What are the most common causes of infertility? If you suspect you might be infertile, when should you seek help? Even then, whom should you consult, and what does an infertility evaluation entail? The treatments available for infertile couples range from simple advice to a bewildering array of medications and new technologies for assisted reproduction. If faced with these choices, would you know what to choose? Then, finally, when should a couple stop infertility treatments, and is adoption a viable option for them when they do?

After reading this book, you'll be in a better position to control your own reproductive destiny. You'll know measures you can take to prevent an infertility problem from ever occurring. Then, if you find you do need the assistance of an infertility expert, you will not only know what to expect, but you will also be able to facilitate your treatment. It's clear that couples who come to an appointment armed with knowledge of their medical, social, and family histories can help their doctors zero in on problem areas.

Postponing Parenthood is not simply a book about infertility. Rather, it's a book that thoroughly and honestly assesses the emotional issue of delayed childbearing. That's what makes it unique. Gale Sloan has done an excellent job of answering many of the questions that I find women have about aging and their ability to conceive. In short, *Postponing Parenthood* provides the information that every couple should have before even beginning to try to become pregnant.

Paul B. Marshburn, M.D.
Division of Reproductive Endocrinology
and Infertility
Department of Obstetrics and Gynecology
University of Texas Southwestern Medical Center
Dallas, Texas

Acknowledgments

To acknowledge the people who helped make this book possible, I would first have to thank Jerome Stern and W. T. Lhamon, two of my writing professors at Florida State University. They showed me that writing is both an art and a discipline, and that it is indeed possible to transform dry medical facts into a story that is entertaining as well as informative. This is my goal whenever I sit down to write.

I'd also like to thank the many women who shared with me their desires, fears, and concerns about delayed childbearing. Their comments helped me to see, over and over again, that women are not only basing decisions that could alter their entire lives on a dearth of information, but they're also often making those decisions based on a great deal of misinformation. I hope this book will help to change that.

I'd especially like to thank Paul Marshburn, M.D., for his tireless enthusiasm for this project, and for his meticulous review of the manuscript for technical accuracy. And finally, I'd like to thank Norma Fox, my editor at Insight Books, and Frank Darmstadt, Assistant Editor, for having the confidence necessary to allow me to turn my idea into reality.

Gale A. Sloan

Contents

INTRODUCTION

How Late to Wait?

If you're thinking about postponing parenthood until after age 30, or even age 35, do you have the information you need to decide how late you can wait?

Deciding to have a child is an important decision, a decision that should be based on *facts*, not on feeling. While you may know that aging carries with it certain risks for infertility, do you know what, exactly, those risks are? For example, are your chances for becoming pregnant at 39 only slightly less than your chances at age 32, or are they cut in half? Also, have you had an illness, or participated in some behavior, that has placed you at risk for becoming infertile before most women your age? What's more, have you given any thought to how the child of older parents differs from the child whose parents are younger? Knowing the answers to these questions could influence your decision about when to try to become pregnant.

Then, once you do begin your quest for parenthood, do you know how to gauge if it's taking too long? Do you know when to consult a doctor, or even whom to consult? And, if you receive an evaluation for infertility, how can you be sure that the doctor is performing the appropriate tests, or giving you the treatment that's most likely to result in a successful pregnancy? An infertility evaluation can be stressful, expensive, and *time-consuming*. Once you've delayed pregnancy, time is not something you have to waste. Scores of women have wasted valuable time, and expended needless emotional energy, by being treated inappropriately for a fertility problem.

If you're thinking about postponing parenthood, you can rest assured that you're not alone. More women than ever are having babies in their 30s, or even 40s, many of them for the first time. Between 1975 and 1987, the rate of first births to women between the ages of 30 and 34 more than doubled, from 8 births to every thousand women in 1975 to 18.4 for every thousand women in 1987. For example, in 1970, 56,728 women aged 30 or greater had their first child. By 1987, this number had ballooned to over 250,000.[1] And, according to the latest figures from the National Center for Health Statistics, the number of first children born to women aged 40 and over *doubled* between 1984 and 1988.[2]

Part of the reason for this increase is that there are simply more women who are age 30 or greater now than ever before. You can thank the post-World War II baby boom for that. But, that's not the sole reason for this increased birth rate. To begin with, women over age 30 having babies for the first time make up a larger percentage of *all* women having babies. Also, more women are now reaching age 30 without ever having had a child, but, when questioned, most respond that they intend to give birth at least once.[3] What's disturbing here is that these women are blindly trusting that they'll be able to get pregnant as soon as they decide they're ready. After years of being taught that preventing pregnancy was the hard part, they've concluded that having children must be easy. Unfortunately, though, for the vast majority of women, this just isn't true. After years of planning and postponing, they end up shocked to discover that becoming pregnant later in life is more difficult than preventing pregnancy.

That doesn't mean that every woman who wants a child should become pregnant at age 22. There are a variety of valid reasons for wanting to delay motherhood. Many women are choosing to marry later, after they've attained advanced degrees, become independent, and launched careers. Even couples who married at a young age didn't necessarily have children at that time. The divorce rate has tripled since 1960; as a result, many of these couples found their plans for childbearing derailed by divorce. Also, couples no longer feel compelled to have children as soon as they marry. They would rather first build a strong, stable relationship with their spouse before adding children to the picture. Still another factor for this boon in late births—a factor that's easy to overlook—is infertility. By postponing pregnancy beyond a certain point, many women sacrifice their ability to conceive quickly. Just because a woman has a baby at age 39 doesn't mean that she waited that late to begin trying to conceive.

It's estimated that, in the late 1980s, over 4 million couples in the United States had difficulty conceiving a child or carrying a child to term, while another 3 million were conclusively sterile.[4] This means that one couple out of every 12 has difficulty conceiving, and, for couples over age 30, the number is as high as one in seven.[5] Medical experts define infertility as an inability to conceive after having intercourse for a year or more without contraception. On the other hand, sterility is the complete inability to conceive.

Not being able to conceive as quickly as you had anticipated can be extremely frustrating, not to mention the fact that it can create havoc with your personal and professional life. For example, if you've chosen to postpone your first pregnancy because of certain career goals or commitments, and you don't conceive about the time you had planned, you could miss out on several key opportunities. This is especially frustrating for achievement-oriented women who have always accomplished everything they've wanted through determination and hard work. Unfortunately, determination and hard work don't guarantee a successful pregnancy.

Another problem is that older couples, because they have delayed having children, often feel under great pressure to conceive in a short period of time. When pregnancy does not result as quickly as they had anticipated, they are left feeling dazed, stressed, and totally helpless—which is not the atmosphere in which you imagined you would conceive your child. It's also second nature to jump to the conclusion that something must be wrong, which may or may not be true.

Some experts feel that doctors give patients the diagnosis of infertility much more often than is warranted, thus generating needless testing and unnecessary treatment.[6] This may be because the criterion for infertility—which is one year of unprotected intercourse without a conception—may be a little too confining. But it's also because more doctors than ever have a financial stake in infertility services. This only makes sense when you consider that the number of births, along with the demand for obstetrical services, declined between 1962 and 1975.[7] As a result, many obstetricians expanded their practices to include infertility—which means that they have a financial interest in treating patients with this problem. It also means that many of the doctors treating women for infertility have not received any advanced training in this most exact science.

A good specialist—when needed—can make the difference between your having a healthy baby or your remaining childless. The problem is knowing when, or whether, treatment is necessary. Hopefully you won't ever need this service. But, if you do, you need to have the appropriate information for making what could be extremely important decisions regarding your reproductive health. It's also a good idea to consider this information when first deciding when to try to conceive. For example, if you know that you're at risk for a problem that could take years to correct, you may decide not to delay until the last minute to begin trying to become pregnant.

The point is, you can't make an intelligent decision about when to have children without having all of the facts—which is where this book can prove invaluable. It will explain how aging affects your ability to conceive and will detail the risks you face if you choose to delay motherhood. Next, it will tell you how to maintain your fertility through those years of delay by minimizing risk factors. Then, once you choose to try to conceive, it will tell you how to maximize your chances for pregnancy. It will also help you identify when something might be wrong, and explain both what a doctor can learn from an infertility workup and what can be done about it. But, above all, it will give you the information you need to make decisions about this part of your life, just as you've made decisions about every other part.

1

The Process of Reproduction

Before we explore the issue of aging and reproduction, you first need to understand at least the basics about the process of reproduction. While the reproductive system may seem like a straightforward series of tubes and passageways, it is, in fact, a complex system of organs—each with its own special function.

A woman's reproductive system consists of the vagina—a tube-shaped canal opening to the outside of the body—and the uterus—a hollow, muscular organ that sits on top of the vagina. The uterus houses the fetus as it develops during pregnancy. Serving as an entryway to the uterus, and also connecting the uterus to the vagina, is a mouthlike structure called the cervix. The next organs of importance are the fallopian tubes, which extend out of the top of the uterus like two horns. These delicate, tubelike organs branch toward the ovaries, where eggs are stored. Just before the fallopian tubes meet the ovaries, the solid structure of the tubes gives way to a fringe of tiny filaments. These flowerlike filaments sweep over the ovary at the time of ovulation, reaching to catch the egg as it springs from its home base. (See Figure 1.)

To function, though, these organs depend on a group of hormones. These hormones are far from static. Rather, they pulsate and change as if participating in a delicate dance: one surges and another falls back in a pattern that repeats itself

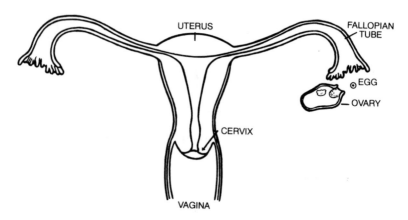

Figure 1.   The female reproductive organs.

every 28 days or so. The first half of the pattern, called the follicular phase, begins on the first day of menstrual bleeding and lasts about 14 days. The hormone FSH, or follicle-stimulating hormone, begins the dance by nudging several immature follicles, each of which contains an egg, inside one or both of your ovaries. The stimulating interest of FSH causes these follicles to grow and begin to mature; however, only one usually develops into a mature egg.

About this same time, the ovaries begin to secrete increasing amounts of an estrogenlike hormone called estradiol. Estradiol stimulates the uterus to produce a thick, rich lining, or endometrium, which will nourish the egg if it becomes fertilized. This hormone also signals the cervix to relax its usual tight-lipped appearance, encouraging it to open wider than usual so that sperm can enter. To further welcome any sperm, the cervix produces an abundance of a rich, clear, elastic mucus. This mucus provides a comfortable, nourishing environment in which the sperm can live until they pass into the uterus and fallopian tubes. The fallopian tube is the most common spot for the egg and sperm to meet.

Then, when everything is ready, the second stage begins. This phase—called the luteal phase—is under the tutelage of the hormone LH, or luteinizing hormone. LH contributes to the maturation of the egg, but its most important role is ovulation itself. Sometime in the middle of the menstrual cycle, LH surges, causing the mature egg to ease out of the comfortable confines of the ovary. The filaments of the fallopian tube grab the traveling egg, and the tube itself begins to undulate, slowly propelling the egg toward the uterus. At the same time, tiny, fingerlike projections, called cilia, which line the inside of the fallopian tube, begin to wave, tickling the egg onward toward its final destination. Thus encouraged, the egg moves forward for the next 12 to 24 hours, making itself available to any interested sperm.

When the egg takes off from the ovary, it leaves behind a kind of shell, called the corpus luteum. The corpus luteum perches at the edge of the ovary, secreting the hormones estradiol and progesterone. These hormones maintain the rich endometrial lining in the uterus, just in case a fertilized egg should arrive. Also, because ovulation has already occurred, these hormones signal the cervix to tighten its relaxed stance and thicken and toughen its mucus; this discourages any late-arriving sperm from entering.

If, after about six days of travel, a fertilized egg arrives in the uterus, the corpus luteum will continue to secrete its hormones until the developing placenta can take over the task. But, if the egg is not fertilized, the corpus luteum quits its post. The levels of estrogen and progesterone plummet, the endometrium sloughs off, and menstruation occurs.

The Male Reproductive System

Men, too, secrete the hormones FSH and LH. However, in them, the levels remain constant. In men, FSH stimulates sperm formation, while LH triggers testosterone production. Testosterone is the hormone that promotes the development of masculine sex characteristics. As far as conception is concerned, the most important aspect of the male system is the production of sperm and the delivery of that sperm into the female's vagina.

Unlike a woman's sexual organs, most of a man's sexual organs are outside his body. These visible organs consist of the penis and the scrotum. The scrotum, or scrotal sack, contains the two organs primarily responsible for the production and maturation of sperm: the testes and the epididymis.

The testes, of which there are two, are small, round organs containing a series of tiny tubules. Under the continual prodding of the hormone FSH, these tubules produce a generous supply of sperm. Once produced, the sperm move up to the epididymis, a tubular organ that sits like a cap on the testes. The epididymis acts as a sort of prep school for the sperm, holding them until they have had time to mature. As that big day approaches, the sperm begin to ease out of the epididymis and into a long, thin tube, or duct. This duct leads the sperm upward, out of the scrotal sack and toward the bladder. The duct doesn't actually enter the bladder; instead, it curves around and joins the urethra, a duct that extends through the penis and out of the body.

During sexual stimulation, the sperm travel farther along the duct, moving quickly away from the epididymis. Along the way, a trio of organs—the seminal vesicles, the prostate gland, and the bulbourethral glands—add fluid and mucus to the band of traveling sperm. This added mixture protects and nourishes the sperm on their journey outside the body. The final product, called semen, propels itself further along the duct until it travels through the penis and out of the body during ejaculation.

Making a Baby

Once the sperm enter the vagina, they begin their battle to make their way up to the fallopian tubes. The first assault against the sperm occurs in the vagina. Normally, the vagina contains acidic fluids that kill sperm. Although the semen contains fluids to help counteract this effect, 90% of the sperm die here, without ever making it any farther. The lucky 10% that make it through the vagina quickly congregate in the welcoming cervix. From here, the most eager sperm move up through the uterus and fan out into each of the fallopian tubes. Usually, only one fallopian tube will contain an egg. Sperm can arrive in the fallopian tubes within 10 minutes of ejaculation; however, many more sperm hang back in the cervix, where they can remain for several days. Protected by the cervical mucus, they break free at intervals and travel up toward the fallopian tubes in search of an egg.

The fact that conception ever takes place seems miraculous when you consider the odds. First of all, the timing has to be fairly precise. If the sperm try to enter the cervix at any time other than during the day or so surrounding ovulation, they will be immediately halted by a wall of thick, impenetrable mucus. Next, even if the timing is perfect, only a few hundred sperm, out of the millions that are ejaculated, make it to the appropriate fallopian tube. Besides the sperm that are immediately killed by the acidic environment of the vagina, others die in the uterus or dart up the wrong fallopian tube. And finally, about 40% of the time, the egg never reaches the fallopian tube. Remember that the fallopian tube has to spread its filaments and catch the egg as it explodes from the ovary. But even with the help of the filaments that fringe the edge of the tube like a catcher's glove, the tube often misses and the egg plummets down into the abyss of the abdomen.

That's why the odds of becoming pregnant in any one month, even when everything is working perfectly, is only about 30%.[1] This means that, for any group of women with normal reproductive ability wanting to become pregnant for the first time, about half of them will become pregnant within five months, and about half of those remaining will become pregnant within the next five months.[2] That leaves a final 25% who take even longer to conceive.

So, as you can see, becoming pregnant can take time, even when everything is in sync. But, many factors can disrupt your, or your partner's, delicately timed reproductive rhythm. These factors range from things you can easily eliminate—such as smoking or douching—to matters requiring medical treatment—such as blocked fallopian tubes. But one factor that can disrupt your ability to conceive is one over which you have no control: aging.

2

Aging and the Reproductive Cycle

Most women know that their reproductive years are limited. After all, people have been talking about a woman's biological clock for some time. Now, though, many women want to know exactly how much time remains before their clocks wind down. But, if they listen to the information portrayed by most of the popular press, they could easily gain the impression that they have years before they need to be concerned. After all, Glenn Close and Bette Midler delivered healthy babies while they were in their 40s, didn't they? That's true, and you might be able to do the same. But don't be misled. Aging definitely affects your ability to conceive, and, if you want to postpone being a parent, you need to know what you're risking.

Determining Reproductive Time Limits

Unfortunately, there are no cut-and-dried numbers to tell you exactly when you will stop being fertile. Researchers have had an idea for years about when a woman's reproductive ability begins to decline, but they have never known exactly. The reason for this is that the information they need to make these predictions is almost impossible to collect in today's society. For example, to determine how fertile women are once they pass the age of 35, researchers might study birth rates for all women in this age group. But the figures derived from this type of study would be less than representative of that population's actual ability to conceive. This is because many couples in that group would be using birth control to keep from becoming pregnant, while other women might choose to terminate a pregnancy. Therefore, the resultant figures would only tell you how many women of a certain age were having babies, not how many have the potential to have children. After all, how do you know if you're able to have a baby until you try to become pregnant?

So that you can understand exactly what your doctor means when he tells you that your time for having children is running out, you need to know on what he's basing his opinion. The foundation for the beliefs concerning how a woman's fertility rate declines with age rests on studies of populations several hundred years old. For example, some of the key populations studied include the Hutterites (a religious group living in the northern United States and Canada in the 1920s and 1930s), Geneva bourgeoisie in the 1600s, Canadian marriages in the early 1700s, and marriages in Normandy in the late 1700s. Now, I know what you're thinking: how can people who lived 300 years ago have any relevance to me? The truth is, though, they do. It was only by reaching back that far in history that researchers could find groups of people who didn't use any form of birth control and, therefore, didn't artificially alter the birth rates. By studying these groups, researchers discovered some valuable information regarding how fertility is affected by a woman's age. Time and again, the groups studied revealed birth rates that suggested that a woman's fertility declines slightly from age 20 to age 30, slips a little more after age 30, and then, after age 35, really drops.[1]

But these statistics aren't without their problems. For example, some researchers have stated that the Hutterites aren't representative of a modern population because, genetically, they most likely had a very high reproductive capacity.[2] On the other hand, as regards all of the groups, if no one was using any form of birth control, the women would no doubt have had numerous children by the time they reached age 35. And, repeated child-bearing in the 1600s and 1700s placed women at considerable risk for developing reproductive abnormalities later in life. This alone could have contributed to the drop in fertility rates for women past age 35. And finally, to be an accurate representation of fertility, one would also have to consider how long the couples had been married. It's pretty much an accepted fact in medical and scientific communities that the longer a couple has been married the less frequently they have sex. So, if all of these groups married at a young age, they might have a decreased chance for having a child by the time they reached their mid to late 30s because they weren't having sex very often.

To overcome these problems (that birth rates dropped simply because of a decreased frequency of sexual intercourse or because of reproductive disorders resulting from previous child-bearing), researchers searched for yet other groups of people to study. This time, they looked for groups that not only didn't use birth control, but also tended to marry later in life. In theory, this would eliminate the risk of the women having developed reproductive disorders because of previous childbearing. And, if they were newlyweds, they most likely were having sex on a regular basis. The scientists found seven such groups, and, when they compiled the resultant data, they discovered that only 9% of women who married between the ages of 25 and 29 remained childless, while 15% of those who married between the ages of 30 and 34 never had children. This figure jumped to 30% for those between the ages of 35 and 39 and, by the time a woman was over age 40, she ran a 64% risk of never having children.[3] These figures, again, suggest that a woman's ability to have a child declines slightly after age 30 and then drops significantly after age 35.

Keep in mind, though, these figures were derived from *historical* populations, not from today's society. The infertility rates discussed in these studies could very well be higher than what would be found in a group of women today. To begin with, the medical care a woman would receive today during pregnancy and during delivery is more likely to prevent any reproductive impairment. Also, medical care today can often treat many conditions that, in the days of the Hutterites, would have interfered with a woman's ability to conceive.

But, it's important that you know about these studies so that you understand the basis for the theories about a woman's biological clock. Until recently, these studies of historical populations were all scientists had on which to base their conclusions about a woman's ability to conceive at a certain age. That's why, in 1982, when the *New England Journal of Medicine* published the results of a study that appeared to finally pinpoint exactly when, and by how much, a woman's ability to have a child decreased with age, the medical community stood up and took notice.[4]

This study was performed by a group of French scientists with an organization called Federation CECOS, which stands for Federation des Centres d'Etude et de Conservation du Sperme Humain, or, loosely translated, the Centers for the Study and Conservation of Human Sperm. In this study, the scientists analyzed the cases of 2193 women whose husbands' semen contained no living sperm; in other words, their husbands were sterile. The women, whose reproductive systems were normal, were being artificially inseminated with sperm donated by someone other than their husbands. Because the women were being artificially inseminated, the timing or frequency of sexual intercourse as a factor in whether or not they became pregnant was eliminated. And, the fact that their husbands were sterile acted as a further control; the only way these women would become pregnant would be through the insemination they received from the donor sperm and not through any sexual activity with their husbands. Therefore, except for age, these women were essentially identical.

The results of the study were significant. The researchers found that a woman's ability to become pregnant began to decline at age 30, and then, by age 35, her ability to become pregnant dropped markedly. To be specific, 74% of the women less than age 31 conceived within 12 insemination cycles. But, only 61% of the women between the ages of 31 and 35 conceived within the same time interval. This number dropped to 54% for women over age 35. In other words, according to this study, a woman's ability to conceive drops by over one-fourth between the ages of 30 and 35. That's startling.

But every study has its faults—and its critics—and this one is no exception. Some have complained that the reported fertility rates are too low because, under most circumstances, artificial insemination has a lower success rate than does normal intercourse.[5] The reasons for this include the possibility that freezing sperm (which is how the sperm used in artificial insemination are preserved until the time of insemination) decreases the sperm's ability to fertilize an egg. Also, because artificial insemination is usually a one-time attempt each month, the correct timing of ovulation is critical. In a normal population, timing is much less important because a couple can have sex over a period of several days.

To remedy these faults, another group of researchers decided to analyze the conception histories of women in a normal population. For this study, they asked a group of women between the ages of 14 and 44 if, during the 3 years before the interview, they had scheduled intercourse in an attempt to become pregnant. What they found seemed to back up the earlier studies. There was little difference in the probability of conception between women in their teens and women in their late 20s. But, the chances of becoming pregnant in any one year dropped for women over age 30. To be specific, about 50% of women less than age 30 conceived in 6 to 7 months. But, the same proportion of women over age 30 had to schedule intercourse for at least 12 months to become pregnant. On the average, women over age 30 who scheduled intercourse to conceive had to wait longer than younger women did before becoming pregnant.[6]

A similar study, but one with slightly different results, used data collected in the 1976 National Survey of Family Growth to calculate the proportion of couples who were continuously married, did not use contraceptives, and did not conceive during the 12 months before the interview. For those between the ages of 20 and 24, only 6.7% did not conceive. This number rose to 10.8% for those aged 25 to 29, to 16.1% for those aged 30 to 34, and to 22.9% for those aged 35 to 39.[7] These figures present a much more optimistic picture of the fertility rates of women in their 30s; however, they still show that fertility rates decline after about age 30 and then continue to slide with age. In fact, researchers at Princeton University estimate that more than 55% of married women between the ages of 40 and 44 have fertility problems.[8]

Why Aging Affects Fertility

By this point, you may be saying, "Okay, I accept the fact that, at age 35, I'm not as fertile as I was at age 20. But why not? I still menstruate, same as always." That's a good question but, again, it's not one that can be answered definitively. However, there are several theories as to why fertility declines with age.

One theory is that aging affects the relationship between the ovaries and certain centers in the brain. The hypothalamus, which is a portion of the brain, and the pituitary gland, which resides in the brain, are key players in the ovulatory cycle. The hypothalamus acts as a sort of foreman, seeing to it that the pituitary gland and, in turn, the ovaries produce enough of the hormones necessary for ovum (egg) maturation and ovulation. But, with age, the hypothalamus may relax its normally assertive posture. Without the boss's constant prodding, the pituitary gland and the ovaries may become lackadaisical and fail to produce their monthly hormone quota. And without an adequate supply of hormones, the eggs can't mature and be released. Along this same line, it's also possible that, even though the hormones may be available, the ovaries are too exhausted from a lifetime of work to respond appropriately. Either way, you don't ovulate as consistently as you did when you were younger.

Another widely accepted reason for the decline of fertility with age is that the eggs contained in the ovary become old and begin to break down. After all, on the day you're born, you have all of the eggs that you're ever going to have. Therefore, every year that you age means that your eggs grow a year older, also. So, you still may ovulate, but the eggs that spring forth are no longer in peak shape. This means that one of two things may happen. First, the eggs may be so structurally altered that they can't even be fertilized. Or, if they are fertilized, they wouldn't develop properly. If this happens, your body would probably slough off the aberrant egg before you even knew you were pregnant.

Another possibility is that, with age, the uterus no longer has the energy to produce, month in and month out, a thick and abundant lining, or endometrium. This is particularly true if the endometrium is diseased in some way, such as from an infection or by a fibroid (a benign growth of fibrous tissue). More often, though, the ovaries fail to produce enough estrogen and progesterone, which causes the uterine lining to be thin or weak. As a result, even if a fertilized egg shows up, the egg can't nestle in for the required months of growth and development. Without the necessary nourishment and support, the egg would, again, simply slough off.

Other theories that researchers have tossed out in an effort to explain a woman's declining fertility revolve around the fact that you've simply been around longer. This means that you've had more time to be exposed to certain environmental toxins, and that you've had a greater chance of contracting an infection or disorder (such as pelvic inflammatory disease or endometriosis) that could play havoc with your reproductive system.

And finally, at least one researcher, William James, feels that one of the main reasons fertility decreases with age is simply that older couples don't have sex as often as do younger couples.[9] After all, how many 40-year-olds have the sexual stamina they did when they were 23?

These are only theories, of course, but each has medical

studies to back it up. When considering the aging of your reproductive system, remember that we're not just talking chronologic age; we're talking *biologic* age. This means how old your organs seem to be, no matter how long they've been around. The aging of your reproductive system is linked more to genetics and the luck of the draw as opposed to whether or not you eat red meat or exercise regularly.

You may have always thought that you'd be able to have children up until the time menopause set in. But, as you can see, that's not true. In fact, most women become infertile as many as 10 years before menopause even starts.[10] Since the average age of menopause in the United States is about age 50, this means that a great number of women become infertile around age 40. And still, these women will continue to ovulate, and continue to menstruate each month, just like normal. They won't have a clue that their biological clocks are winding down unless, of course, they try to become pregnant.

But, aging doesn't affect just women. It affects men, too—just not as dramatically or as rapidly. Many researchers believe that a 50- to 54-year-old man has about 73% the level of fertility he had in his early 20s.[11] However, other researchers think that men over the age of 40 have only a 30% chance of impregnating a woman within 6 months as compared to a man in his early 20s.[12] This means that, if you're in your late 30s, and your husband is in his 40s, your risk of having subnormal fertility is just that much greater.

Aging and Fertility Rates: The Bottom Line

Now, before you decide that you have to start trying to get pregnant immediately, or before you give up all hope of ever becoming pregnant, consider this: sterility, or extreme infertility, isn't something that occurs the day after your 35th birthday. Rather, infertility is a process that occurs over time.[13] This means that there are a number of years during which you still have the ability to become pregnant, but it will just take you longer to conceive than it would have when you were in your 20s.

Remember also that all of these statistics are based on a woman's ability to conceive within a 12-month period of time. This alone brands many women who will ultimately have children as infertile. For example, a study of women in rural English parishes compared the age of a woman at the time of her marriage to whether or not she had any children. The results of the study agreed with earlier studies as to the pattern of sterility due solely to the process of aging.[14] In addition, the study found that 23% of the women who married between the ages of 20 and 24 failed to have a live birth within the first 2 years of marriage. By today's standards, all of these women would have been classified as infertile. And yet, only 4.6% of these women never had a child.[15] In another British study, 80% of women had a conception that later ended in a birth after one year of trying. But, 39 months later, 91% of the women had conceived.[16]

This shows that using 12 months as the cutoff point between whether a woman is fertile or not may be a little too stringent. Granted, many women who can't conceive within a 12-month period of time are either sterile or have a medical problem that prevents them from becoming pregnant. But many more women are still capable of conceiving. Even among women who are exceptionally fertile, some experts estimate that it takes an average of 8 months to conceive. They further estimate that at least 14% of this same highly fertile group may take more than a year to conceive.[17] When you combine this information with the fact that a woman becomes less fertile as she grows older, you can see that becoming pregnant may simply take time.

A study published in the *New England Journal of Medicine* in 1983 clearly illustrates this. In this study, the researchers followed 1145 infertile couples over a period of 2 to 7 years to determine how often pregnancy occurred despite treatment. The results showed that, of the 597 couples who received treatment, 41% became pregnant. But, of the 548 couples who received no treatment, 35% became pregnant anyway. Further-more, of the couples who received treatment, 31% of the preg-nancies occurred more than 3 months after the last medical treatment.[18]

This is not to say that you should never seek treatment for infertility. Doctors are able to do remarkable things, and many women who would have never stood a chance of becoming pregnant are delivering healthy babies. Rather, it's meant to say that you need to allow yourself time. If you're over age 30, and you're trying to figure out when to start a family, consider that it may take you more than a year to conceive. No matter what your age, if you've been trying for a year without success, then you may want to consider having a medical evaluation to deter-mine if there is an identifiable, and treatable, cause for the delay. And, if you're over age 35, it's a good idea to wait no longer than about six months; that way, if there is a diagnosable cause for your infertility, you'll be able to receive treatment before too much more time ticks away. At the same time, though, don't let that year, or six-month, marker throw you into a fit of despair. While you need to be realistic about your increased risk of hav-ing a problem, realize also that, just because you're older, con-ception may take longer.

Also keep your plan to postpone parenthood in perspec-tive. Your wish may be to complete school, advance in your career, or simply save some money before having children. If so, you need to weigh carefully the benefits of these goals—which you may be able to achieve only by postponing parenthood—with the risks of having a delayed conception, or no conception, at a later date.

John Bongaarts, senior associate with the Center for Policy Studies of the Population Council, has concluded that delaying childbearing may not be all that grim. He estimates that if a woman is now 25 to 29 years old, and wants to postpone having a baby by 5 years, then her risk of infertility only increases by 4%. He carries this further to say that, if she's now 30 to 34 years old, and wants to postpone for 5 years, then her risk of infertility will increase 10% above what it currently is.[19]

I must say that Mr. Bongaarts, among all of the researchers, is one of the more optimistic regarding a woman's ability to conceive at later ages. Don't forget that a significant amount of research strongly suggests that a woman's reproductive ability declines after age 30 and then drops significantly after age 35. But, as he has so succinctly stated, most of life's decisions involve a balancing of risks and benefits. This means balancing the risks of being infertile with the benefits of waiting to have a baby.

3

The Risks of a Postponed Pregnancy

Doctors used to roll their eyes and groan when they saw a woman over age 35 pregnant with her first child. A "high-risk pregnancy" they'd call it, as they prepared for a succession of complications, beginning a few weeks after conception and continuing through the labor and delivery process. For the most part, this attitude of foreboding has changed as more women have safely and successfully completed pregnancies after the "advanced" age of 35. Some of the complications doctors worried about as going hand-in-hand with a mother's older age have turned out *not* to be linked to age, after all. What's more, women over age 30 are often more inclined to seek medical care, both early in the pregnancy and whenever any sign of a problem occurs. But the news isn't all good. You'll still face several risks if you delay having your baby until late in your reproductive life.

Risks after You First Conceive

You need to know that—simply because of your age—you're at risk for suffering two major complications during the first few weeks of pregnancy. The first is your risk for having a miscarriage. The second is your risk for discovering that the child you conceived has a chromosomal abnormality.

Miscarriage

When making your decision about when to start your family, you need to consider that, the older you are, the greater is your risk for having your pregnancy end in miscarriage. In fact, women past age 35 are nearly twice as likely to suffer a miscarriage as are women in their mid to late 20s. Consider these figures: a woman between the ages of 25 and 29 has only about a 10% chance of having a miscarriage. Up until age 34, this risk increases just slightly, to 11.7%. But, by the time a woman is between the ages of 35 and 39, she has a 17.7% chance of having a miscarriage. Then, by the time she's 40, her risk of having her pregnancy end in miscarriage is up to 33.8%.[1]

Some of the reasons for this increased miscarriage rate are the same as the reasons for a decreased fertility rate. One reason is that older eggs may not develop properly after fertilization. As was discussed previously, a mother's body often rejects abnormal embryos. The body's desire to create only a normal fetus is so great that it's estimated that 65% of the pregnancies involving a fetus with Down's syndrome, and even more of those involving other chromosomal abnormalities, end in miscarriage.[2] If this sloughing off of an abnormal embryo occurs early enough in the development process, you may never even know that you'd been pregnant. But, if it occurs later, you would have been aware of your pregnancy, so that the sloughing off process becomes a recognizable miscarriage.

Another reason for this increased miscarriage rate in older mothers is that the uterus may be less able to support a growing embryo. After a certain age, women are more likely to have a hormonal abnormality that would impair the ability of the uterus to maintain a pregnancy. Also, women over age 35 are more likely to have a uterine fibroid (a benign growth in the uterus), which could interfere with the developing fetus. Finally, by the time you reach age 35, you have a greater chance of having a disease, such as atherosclerosis or diabetes, which could cause poor circulation to the uterus and trigger a miscarriage.

Whatever the reason, dealing with the emotional aspects of miscarriage isn't easy, especially if you've been trying for months, or years, to get pregnant. Therefore, when you're planning for pregnancy, you need to consider your age and then consider that your first pregnancy may not end in a live birth. The odds are still good that it will, but it's better to be aware of this risk and maybe allow yourself a little more time, than to wait until the last second to conceive and then have your last-chance pregnancy end in miscarriage.

Fetal Chromosomal Abnormalities

The second big risk you'll have to face if you get pregnant later in life is that you may conceive a child with a chromosomal abnormality. This risk rises in direct relation to a woman's age—so much so that most doctors routinely encourage all pregnant patients older than age 35 to undergo tests to screen for such abnormalities.

Down's syndrome—also called trisomy 21—is perhaps the most recognized genetic abnormality of children of older mothers. To understand why this disorder occurs, you first need to know that an egg contains 23 pairs of chromosomes (46 chromosomes), whereas a sperm contains only 23 unpaired chromosomes. As the egg prepares to be fertilized by the sperm, it splits its 23 pairs of chromosomes in two. It discards one set, and waits with the other set of 23 unpaired chromosomes. When the sperm pierces the egg's outer shell, it matches its 23 unpaired chromosomes to the 23 unpaired chromosomes in the egg, thus creating a new, unique set of chromosomes. The problem develops because, with older eggs, some of the chromosomes have deteriorated and tend to stick together. This is a particular problem for the 21st chromosome. Therefore, when the egg attempts to unpair each of its chromosomes, the 21st paired chromosome sometimes refuses to split in two. As a result, after fertilization, there is a normal set of pairs for each chromosome except for number 21, which now has not just a pair, but three chromosomes; thus the name, *trisomy 21* ("tri" meaning "three"), or *Down's syndrome.*

Down's syndrome, sometimes referred to as mongoloidism, usually causes the baby to be born mentally retarded. Although the severity of the disorder varies, children with Down's syndrome usually live into adulthood; however, their mental abilities don't progress much beyond those of a 5- or 6-year-old.[3] Besides having mental deficiencies, children with Down's syndrome are likely to have physical abnormalities as well, including malformations of the heart or intestinal tract.

For women aged 23, only 1 fetus out of 1429 will be afflicted with Down's syndrome, while only 1 out of 500 will have some other type of chromosomal abnormality. By the time a woman is 30 years of age, the risk for Down's syndrome increases to 1 out of 952 births, while the risk for any chromosomal abnormality is 1 out of 385. Age 35 sees the risk for Down's syndrome jump to 1 out of 378 fetuses, with the risk for any chromosomal abnormality increasing to 1 out of 192. Then, by age 40, the risk for having a Down's syndrome child is 1 out of 106, and the risk for any type of chromosomal abnormality is 1 out of 66.[4]

Fathers older than age 40 also contribute to the risk for having a child with a congenital abnormality (birth defect).[5] Most researchers believe that men contribute the chromosome that causes Down's syndrome 20 to 25% of the time, and that men over age 40 are at higher risk for causing about a dozen other uncommon genetic diseases.[6]

There's no question that these statistics look grim. But the good news is that even if the risk for Down's syndrome is 1 out of a hundred, as it is for women aged 40, there's still a 99% chance that the baby *won't* have Down's syndrome. The second bit of good news is that tests exist to screen women for many of the possible genetic abnormalities.

The first step to see if you're especially at risk is to examine your own family history. Many abnormalities run in families, and if a certain abnormality runs in your or your husband's family, you could be at risk for passing that abnormality along to your child.

As far as diagnostic tests go, a relatively simple test used to screen for several birth defects, including neural tube defects, is a blood test called AFP, which stands for alpha-fetoprotein. AFP is a protein produced by the fetus and passed into the mother's blood. To perform the test, a blood sample is drawn sometime between the 15th and 20th weeks of pregnancy. If the value is too high, it could mean that the fetus has some type of defect in his spine or his brain. In this instance, the doctor would probably follow the test with an ultrasound to check for any structural abnormalities. If the level is too low, it could mean that the fetus has a chromosomal abnormality, such as Down's syndrome. If this occurs, the doctor would no doubt recommend an amniocentesis for a more exact assessment.

Amniocentesis remains the favored test for diagnosing chromosomal abnormalities. Most doctors recommend performing the procedure on any pregnant woman aged 35 or older. They feel that, by this age, the risk of having a genetic disorder outweighs the risk of the procedure.[7] Performed during the 15th or 16th week of pregnancy, this test involves inserting a needle through the abdomen and into the uterus and removing a sample of the amniotic fluid surrounding the fetus. The fetal cells contained in the fluid are then analyzed for chromosomal abnormalities. Although relatively safe, the test isn't without complications. Most of the complications are fairly mild, such as vaginal bleeding and fluid leakage; however, miscarriage does occur as a result of the test in about 1 out of every 200 tests.[8]

Besides the disadvantage of having to wait two to three weeks to receive your test results, you'll also be well into your second trimester before you can have the test performed. This means that if you choose to terminate the pregnancy based on the results of the test, you would have to admit yourself to the hospital for an abortion by chemical induction. This causes your uterus to go into contractions and expel the fetus. Although this type of an abortion is safe, it is, needless to say, extremely stressful.

A test that can be performed earlier than the amniocentesis, and that can reveal much of the same information, is chorionic villus sampling, or C.V.S. This test, which is performed between the 8th and 10th weeks of pregnancy, involves the removal of a tiny amount of tissue from what will eventually become the placenta. To remove the tissue, the doctor may insert an instrument either through the vagina or through the abdomen. Because both the placenta and the fetus develop from the same fertilized egg, these cells will mirror any chromosomal abnormalities of the fetus.

The advantage of this procedure over the amniocentesis is that it can be done weeks earlier. This means that, if there is an abnormality and the parents choose to terminate the pregnancy, it can be done quickly and easily in a doctor's office or clinic. Also, because the test is performed before most women show any outward signs of pregnancy, they have the option of keeping the fact of their pregnancy private until test results are available. Another advantage is that the results are available in days instead of weeks, which means less time sitting around biting your nails.

The test isn't perfect, however. Chorionic villus sampling causes more than 1 out of every 100 women to have a miscarriage, which is twice the risk as from an amniocentesis. Also, based on the results of several recent studies, some doctors feel C.V.S. may actually *cause* birth defects in a small number of babies. Specifically, according to some statistics, babies born to women who have had C.V.S. may have a higher incidence of a particular rare malformation, involving missing or stubby fingers and toes, and sometimes a shortened tongue and an underdeveloped jaw. The reason behind these malformations isn't clear, although some have speculated that it may result if the C.V.S. procedure causes a tiny hemorrhage in the placenta, interrupting blood supply to the fetus.

Because all the data have yet to be evaluated, experts aren't certain as to the actual incidence of these malformations. However, Dr. Barbara Burton of the Humana Michael Reese Hospital in Chicago told the *New York Times* that, based on data from a workshop of the National Institutes of Health, anywhere from 1 in 200 to 1 in 1000 babies born to women who have had C.V.S. will have the defects.[9]

Conversely, not all doctors agree that these birth defects can be blamed on C.V.S. For example, Dr. Joseph Schulman, director of the Genetics and I.V.F. Institute in Fairfax, Virginia, said that, based on data from more than 50,000 C.V.S. procedures worldwide, there was no increased frequency of limb malformations with C.V.S. Dr. Schulman maintained that C.V.S. is safe, and that those same birth defects can be found in babies born to women who never had the procedure.[10]

Unfortunately, once again, there is no clear choice as to the best procedure. When the time comes to choose, you'll simply need to evaluate all the pros and cons of each procedure and make the choice that's best for you.

What if you would never choose to terminate a pregnancy, regardless of the results of a chromosomal study? Should you still undergo one of these procedures? The choice is yours, of course, but keep in mind that such a test can still provide valuable information. For example, knowing in advance that a child will be born with some type of an abnormality would allow you to prepare emotionally for the birth and to make any necessary arrangements for caring for the child at home. Furthermore, because these children often have special medical needs, the information would also allow the doctor to gather all of the equipment and personnel necessary to ensure that the child's needs would be met from the moment of delivery.

Medical Risks during the Pregnancy

Once you pass these first two hurdles, you're still not home free. As your pregnancy continues, there are other complications that you may have to address.

Hypertension

The most common, and the most serious, complication you may encounter if you have a child after age 35 is high blood pressure, or pregnancy-induced hypertension. In fact, about one-third of all pregnant women over age 35 develop hypertension as a direct result of their being pregnant.[11] Part of the reason for this is age alone; even without the added stress of pregnancy, a woman over age 35 has a greater chance of having high blood pressure even before becoming pregnant than does a younger woman.

While high blood pressure may not seem like much of a problem, it can, indeed, be quite serious and actually lead to the death of the fetus or convulsions in the mother. Needless to say, if you develop high blood pressure while you're pregnant, you'll need to see your doctor more often, and you'll need to be careful to follow his advice.

Diabetes

Another complication that occurs more often in older mothers is diabetes mellitus. As you may already know, diabetes is a metabolic disorder resulting from a deficiency of insulin. Without enough insulin, your body can't properly use the glucose, or sugar, that's available.

During pregnancy, diabetes often manifests itself in women who, under normal conditions, wouldn't have any symptoms of the disease. But, the stress of pregnancy pushes the latent diabetes into the open. In these situations, the diabetes usually disappears after the baby is born. However, during the pregnancy, it's still very much present and requires strict monitoring and control. Developing diabetes during pregnancy can mean that you have a greater likelihood of developing pregnancy-induced hypertension or other complications.

Although statistics vary, a woman over the age of 35 who is pregnant with her first child has a risk for developing diabetes that is about three times greater than that for a younger woman.

If the same woman has been pregnant before, her risk increases to four times. Furthermore, women older than 38 have as much as eight times the risk for developing diabetes than do younger women.[12]

Risks to the Infant

For years, a doctor's greatest concerns when caring for a pregnant woman past the age of 35 have centered around the risks facing the fetus. Even today, your doctor may warn you—and perhaps even scare you—about some of these risks. So that, once you're pregnant, you don't spend months fretting over the health of your fetus, you need to learn what the real risks are. Much new research has discounted the risks long thought linked to the mother's age.

Perinatal Mortality

Doctors have long thought that the main risk women older than 35 having babies for the first time faced was having their babies stillborn or having their babies die from complications shortly after birth. The medical term for this is "perinatal mortality." But, contrary to this long-held medical belief, recent studies have shown that this risk does *not* increase just because of a woman's age. Rather, it seems that it's the severity of certain medical problems, such as hypertension or diabetes, and not the age of the mother, that chiefly affects the health of the fetus.[13]

As an example, consider a study that compared the pregnancies of 1000 women younger than 35 to the pregnancies of 1000 women over 35. The researchers specifically examined how many women in each age group had babies who died either before or shortly after birth. What they found was that 47 of the women over 35 had babies who died, while only 28 of the women younger than 35 had the same complication. Looking at these statistics alone, it would seem that the incidence of perinatal mortality increases as the mother's age increases. But this is not the case.

When the researchers took the study one step further and excluded all of the women who had high blood pressure, they discovered that the number of women who lost babies was the same for each age group.[14] These results are even more encouraging when you consider that, as medical care for both mothers and infants becomes more sophisticated, the number of infants who die should decrease even more. The most recent statistics available indicate that this is, in fact, the case.

From 1968 to 1970, the perinatal mortality rate for infants of women over 35 was 72 per 1000 live births. From 1971 to 1974, the rate decreased to 14 per 1000 live births.[15] To bring these figures more up-to-date, a study in 1983 of over 1000 pregnant women over 35 found that the women in the study, even though they were considered "at risk" because of their age, had no more babies who were stillborn or who died shortly after birth than did younger women. The researchers concluded that these positive findings were due to the expert medical care that women, and their babies, were now able to receive.[16]

The fact you shouldn't ignore, though, is that hypertension and diabetes significantly increase the risk for perinatal mortality. And, as you already know, aging increases your risk for developing these complications when you become pregnant. But, rather than deter you from becoming pregnant, this information should simply reinforce the need for expert medical care beginning the moment you know you're pregnant.

Small Size

Another risk the infant faces if his mother is older than 35 relates to his size—either smaller or larger than normal. On the one hand, a recent study of close to 4000 women, the results of which were published in the *New England Journal of Medicine*, showed that women aged 35 and over were 30% more likely to have a baby that weighed less than $5\frac{1}{2}$ pounds.[17] Having a baby this small means more than that the child needs to gain weight. It means that he's starting life one step behind.

Then, at the other extreme, are studies suggesting that older mothers are much more likely to have babies that are larger than normal.[18] This frequently occurs in women who have diabetes; however, in these instances, it occurred in older women, regardless of whether or not they had diabetes. Having a large baby can make for a difficult vaginal delivery, which, in turn, increases your risk for having a cesarean-section. Even if a doctor can coax a baby through a vaginal delivery, the baby has an increased risk for being injured. After all, the pelvic cavity is only so wide, and squeezing a larger-than-normal baby through a small opening is a setup for injury.

Risks in Labor and Delivery

Finally, the last area of your pregnancy that we need to address is that of labor and delivery. Once again, your doctor may warn you about the risks you'll face during the birth process because of your age. And again, some of these aren't worth worrying about. Following are what you basically need to know about your risks in delivering a child at a later age.

Premature Labor

Doctors have long thought that women over age 35 had a greater risk for delivering their babies prematurely. But, the facts aren't exactly clear as to whether this is or isn't a risk related to a woman's age. Some studies have shown that older women do tend to have their babies prematurely.[19] However, other, larger studies have shown that older women don't go into labor prematurely any more often than younger mothers do.[20,21] So, just be aware of these inconsistent results before you let someone scare you about your risk for delivering too soon.

Prolonged Labor

Another risk that older mothers may or may not face is that of a prolonged labor. Many doctors feel that women having their babies at an older age are more likely to have a prolonged labor. But, although some studies have supported this theory, other more recent and larger studies have not shown this to be the case.[22] So, again, don't let the thought of a long labor cloud your decision-making process.

Cesarean Section

There is one risk that remains consistent from study to study, and that's the mature pregnant woman's risk for having a cesarean section (C-section). This is especially true for women having their first child.[23]

Just why this risk occurs isn't clear, but the fact that it happens is irrefutable. One sizable study showed that the C-section rate in women having their first baby after the age of 35 was double that in women aged 20 to 25.[24] Women who had hypertension or diabetes had an even greater chance of having a C-section. But in these instances, the mother's age wasn't an issue. When hypertension or diabetes was involved, the C-section rate was the same regardless of whether the woman was over or under 35.

No researcher has been able to make a connection as to why older women seem to undergo more C-sections than younger women do. The logical reason would be that these patients had age-related complications of pregnancy that necessitated the procedure. However, this hasn't been the case. Some researchers feel that this high rate for C-sections occurs because doctors are more cautious when dealing with pregnant women over 35. They might feel that women of this age can't tolerate a long labor, or they may worry about a complication occurring. As a result, the doctors may stop the labor process and order a C-section sooner than they would if the women were younger.

Therefore, once you become pregnant, you may want to quiz your doctor about his philosophy regarding the ability of women your age to deliver vaginally. If he feels that older mothers, as long as they're in good physical shape and the fetus is in no danger, should be able to deliver a baby vaginally, then you may have found the doctor for you. But, if he says otherwise, you may want to reconsider your choice.

Other Complications

Finally, some studies have shown that older mothers tend to have babies that have low Apgar scores at birth.[25] Apgar scores are used to rate an infant's overall condition at birth. The scoring system assigns a numerical value to the infant's respiratory effort, muscle tone, color, heart rate, and reflexes. The lower the score, the greater the infant's need for resuscitation efforts. Although having a baby with a low Apgar score has long been linked to the mother's age, a recent study of close to 4000 women published in the *New England Journal of Medicine* found that there was no evidence that this was true.[26]

Long-Term Risks to the Mother

Delaying pregnancy past age 30 also increases your risk for developing breast cancer at a later date. For example, a woman who has her first child before age 18 has about one-third the risk for developing breast cancer as does a woman having her first child after age 34. Not having any children also increases a woman's risk for developing breast cancer; however, the risk here is less than the risk faced by a woman having her first child after age 34.[27] So, if you do have a baby after age 34, this is just one more reason for you to be religious about obtaining annual mammograms and performing monthly breast self-examinations.

The Final Word on Pregnancy after Age 35

By now you may be feeling rather mortal: you've learned that, as you age, your eggs begin to decay, your hormone levels drop, and you may have a reduced chance for delivering a child vaginally. But don't forget the other side of the coin. With proper prenatal care, you have as much of a chance of delivering a healthy baby as does a younger woman.[28] This is especially true if you maintain your ideal body weight. (Some researchers have found that women who were obese were much more likely to develop complications, including hypertension and diabetes.[29])

It's true that, with age, you have a much greater risk of developing complications with your pregnancy. But don't forget that treatment exists for most of these complications. And don't become too obsessed by the changes that are occurring in your body. Keep them in mind, but remember, too, the changes that have occurred in your life that will make you a better parent. Most older parents are more mature, more financially secure, and more willing to settle down to the business of child rearing. Your life experiences will no doubt help you create a caring, nurturing, and instructive environment in which a child can thrive. So don't curse your body for growing old. Rather, expect the changes that are inevitable and learn how to control your risk for infertility. These are the first steps toward successfully postponing your career as a parent.

4

The Child of Older Parents

Now that we've discussed how age will affect your ability to conceive, and your ability to deliver a healthy baby, let's consider one more thing—the effect your age will have on your child. In other words, how will your being an older parent influence the development of your child?

A few studies have revealed some interesting physical differences that may appear in late-born children. For example, some researchers have suggested that the children of older mothers have a higher incidence of fine motor problems. Another study published in the *New England Journal of Medicine* found that older mothers tend to have children who are left-handed[1]; however, other researchers have disputed this claim.[2] Furthermore, a national survey of children found that children of older mothers tend to have higher IQs than do children of younger mothers.[3] Although interesting, these factors don't seem to be any cause for concern. On the other hand, the emotional differences found in late-born children are an entirely different story.

Before we discuss these differences, you need to bear several facts in mind. The first is that the children born to older parents are still in the minority. It's easy to overlook this fact because, according to many couples, "everyone" they know is delaying childbearing. So, they rationalize, even though they're older than what's been considered normal for having children in the past, a new "normal" is evolving. They therefore conclude that the friends their children will make are likely to have parents who are older, too. But this isn't necessarily the case. According to United States birth statistics, in 1987, 250,000 babies were born to women between the ages of 35 and 39. That's a large number of babies, true. But, the total number of babies born during that same period equaled 3.8 million.[4] So, as you can see, the vast majority of children are still born to parents younger than age 35.

Another point to remember is that, contrary to popular belief, this generation is not the first to postpone parenthood. During the Depression, for example, many couples delayed marriage because of financial reasons. Then World War II broke out, and even more couples had to delay both marriage and childbearing. So, when the war ended, couples started to marry and have children in great numbers. And the sharpest increase in birth rates was to women over 35.

The children born during that era are adults now, and they have a lot to say about what it was like to grow up a child of older parents. In light of the fact that so many couples today seem to be delaying childbearing, sociologist Monica Morris of California State University was particularly interested in what this group of people had to say. Therefore, she selected 22 adults whose parents were older than average when they were born; the mothers' age at their birth ranged from 35 to 46, while their fathers were anywhere from 35 to 52 when they were born. Dr. Morris then quizzed these participants at length as to how their lives were affected by their parents' ages. (The complete results of Dr. Morris's study are published in the book *Last Chance Children: Growing Up with Older Parents*, Columbia University Press, 1988.) Similarly, Andrew L. Yarrow interviewed 70 adult children of older parents, and surveyed many others, for his book, *Latecomers: Children of Parents Over 35* (The Free Press, 1991).

Although neither Dr. Morris's study, nor Mr. Yarrow's interview group, had a control group, the responses of these adult children of older parents, when discussing the pros and cons of their childhood, were surprisingly similar. For this reason, their responses merit attention. The information presented here may alter your decision as to when to have children; then again, it may not. Either way, it could open your eyes to problems that may crop up after your children arrive. And if you're aware that a problem may arise, not only will you notice it as soon as it develops, you'll be ready with possible solutions.

Low Parental Energy Level

A common complaint of all of the children of older parents was that their parents didn't play with them the way their friends' parents, who were younger, played with their children. The men, especially, felt deprived because their fathers didn't play sports or roughhouse with them the way they would have liked. Almost all of these adults said they wished they'd had younger parents, parents who would have taken them canoeing or camping, or who would have at least been more interested in throwing around a football. Most remembered being envious of their classmates because their classmates had younger parents.

It's a fact that, as people age, they don't have the energy they did when they were younger. In addition, when people are older, they lose the desire to be as active. Somehow, when you're 45, running around and sweating may not have as strong an appeal as it did when you were 25. Regardless, children need to have parents who are physically active. According to some psychologists, children who have fathers who aren't very playful don't relate to their peers as well as do the children whose parents are more physically active.[5] There's just something about parents rolling around on the floor and being childish with their child that's an important part of development.

Of course, you may feel that now, at age 35 or 40, you have as much energy as you ever did. But, we're not talking about *now*; we're talking about 10 or 15 years from now. That's when your child will be full of energy and will want you to chase him around the yard or play relay games. What will your energy level be like then, when you're 50? Furthermore, when you're entering your 60s, will you be up to weathering the emotional ups and downs that will be a part of living with a child going through the trials and tribulations of adolescence?

An obvious key here is that, if you want to delay childbearing, you must work at keeping yourself in the best physical shape possible—both for your sake as well as your child's. There's really no excuse for not exercising and trying to retain as much of your youthful energy as possible. Of course, no matter how hard you work at preserving youth, the infirmities of age will eventually take over. Exactly when that occurs will depend to a large degree on your family history and your particular genes. You can, however, work on postponing the inevitable. Just two or three extra years of being physically active could make a world of difference both to your child's development and his memories of his childhood.

Besides needing to be physically active, children also need to participate in the same kinds of activities in which their friends participate. For example, time and again, the adult children of older parents stated that they had wanted desperately to take camping vacations like their friends took rather than the luxury vacations that they went on with their older parents. Even though they may have realized that a trip to Europe was a privilege, what they really wanted to be doing was sleeping on the ground and toasting marshmallows.

If the time does arrive when you just aren't able to be as physically active as your child would like, there are alternatives to sprinting up the path to an early heart attack. For one thing, you can be an active spectator. For example, if your child were to play little league baseball, you could make sure that you'd be at every game possible. The time and attention that you'll devote to your child will be as, or even more, important than your actual physical participation. Also, if your child wants to camp and, by this time, you've had three back operations and can't possibly participate, then you could see to it that your child gets the opportunity to camp some other way. This could be by arranging for a friend or relative to take him, or by encouraging him to join an outdoor group. Even if you couldn't actually go on the trip, you could help with the planning and preparations before the trip, and make yourself available to listen to the stories after the trip.

Furthermore, you could find activities that you and your child could do together that wouldn't involve an endurance sport. For example, you could take trips to museums or zoos, or go fishing together. You could also become involved in school activities with your child. Finally, you could see to it that your child will have other people available who could actively participate if you weren't able to. This might be through relatives, church groups, school associations, or neighbors.

The most important thing, overall, is the time you will have available to spend with your child. The adult children of older parents who seemed to feel the most deprived described their parents as desiring to watch television or read the newspaper rather than play. As you can see, that's more than lack of physical participation; that's lack of all participation.

Missed Out on Childhood

Another frequent complaint of these adult children of older parents is that they felt that their parents' older ages forced them to mature too early, that they became "little adults" instead of children. They stated that, as children, they had difficulty relating to children their own age and that they related better to adults.

Part of the reason for this, again, is that older parents tend to be less playful; they tend to discourage childish behavior and to emphasize conversation and more adult activities. Also, when parents are older, their friends, too, are older. And, if these friends didn't also delay childbearing, their children would either be grown or at least significantly older than the child in question. Consequently, at parties or get-togethers, the child of an older parent is either left alone or is forced to associate with adults. Another consequence of their not feeling comfortable around other children is that they tended to spend their free time in solitary pursuits, such as reading or drawing. Of course, there's nothing wrong with these pursuits, but children need a balance. If they're not comfortable being with other children, not only will they miss out on a significant part of their childhood, they'll also fail to develop some very necessary social skills.

Once again, this isn't an insurmountable problem. You will need to be aware of it, though, and you'll need to make an effort to see that your child will have the chance to be a child. Naturally, most of your friends, and probably even your neighbors, are going to be about your same age and have a similar financial status. So, your child may feel somewhat "set apart" from his friends—not just because you're older, but also because you live in a different section of town from many of his peers. If you end up having a child when you're older, you could help your child enjoy his childhood by making an effort to get acquainted with the parents of your child's friends. You could also participate in church groups or school programs where you would meet other adults who have children the same age as your child. As a result, when you did socialize with these people, your child would have company his own age.

Another option would be to see to it that your child spent a significant amount of his after-school time with children his own age. You could accomplish this by inviting other children over to your house for meals or sleep-overs. All of these suggestions take time and energy, to be sure; but remember, it will be important for your child to feel comfortable with children his own age, and that he feel comfortable simply being a child.

Embarrassed by Parents' Age

Most children don't become aware that their parents are any different from anyone else's parents until they reach school age. In some cases, they don't become aware of their parents' ages until they're teenagers. According to one child of an older parent, "I don't think I became aware that my parents were older till my late teens. I always thought they were the same age as everybody else's parents. When I was 10, my mother was 50, but I saw her as 35. It was almost a shock to realize she was 40 years older than I was. When her 55th birthday came around, my friends said, 'Are you kidding?'"[6]

Keep in mind that most children want to be just like their peers, and fitting in includes having parents that are the same ages as their friends' parents. The fact that you'll be older than the parents of most of your child's friends will make you, and your child, stand out. With gray hair and wrinkles, you'll look different, and you'll probably dress differently than the younger parents, too. Even your taste in music will be different.

Many of the adult children of older parents related incidents when their parents were mistaken for their grandparents. The children were either embarrassed themselves, or they felt sad and ashamed for their parents.

Of course, you can't control this entirely. You're going to show signs of age, there's no doubt about it. But you can make an effort to keep current on what's new in fashion, music, etc. Even if you don't participate, you'll at least be aware. You can also improve the situation by not lying about your age. Lying about your age—or simply trying to hide your age by not discussing it—will make the child feel that there's something shameful about being older. In turn, this will only make him more self-conscious and embarrassed about having older parents. Also, if you lie about your age, your child will know. Even if he doesn't discern a difference between your appearance and the appearance of his friends' parents, he'll eventually learn the truth, and then he'll feel betrayed.

A better course is to be open and honest with your child from the beginning. Don't make an issue of your age, but don't hide it either. If you're comfortable with your age, your child will most likely be comfortable with it also. You can also look on this as an opportunity to instill in your child the awareness that there are qualities and virtues that are much more important, and much more enduring, than a person's physical appearance.

Generation Gap

Another problem with having your child late in life, especially if you're in your 40s when you give birth, is that the child often ends up feeling that he's missed a generation. After all, if you give birth in your 40s, you may be closer to the age of your child's friends' grandparents instead of his parents.

This creates two problems. The first is that the child ends up feeling that his parents are too old to understand what it's like to be a child or a teenager. And, let's face it, if 40 years will have passed since you experienced that first rush of hormones, you could have trouble relating to the sexual angst of your teenage child. Almost all of these adult children of older parents stated that they had had difficulty talking to their parents about their problems and concerns; they simply felt that their parents were "too old" to understand.

Another problem is that the children of older parents may end up looking upon their parents more as grandparents than parents. If you will be close to a generation older than the parents of your child's friends, then your values may be different than the values of those younger parents—which are the values against which your child's peers will be rebelling. As a result, the teenagers of older parents won't rebel against their parents. While you may look upon this as a positive result—after all, who wants to put up with a rebellious teenager?—it may, in reality, have negative consequences. The rebellious teenage years are an important "rite of passage" for a child. That's the time when young adults pull away from their parents and establish an identity and value system of their own.

Again, though, solutions exist. First, let's realize that many teenage children aren't comfortable talking with their parents about their personal problems, regardless of how old, or how young, their parents are. You can help ensure that your child will feel comfortable talking with you when he's a teenager by being an empathetic and supportive listener throughout your child's life. This is especially important if there will be a significant age gap between you and your child.

But, even if you try your best, there may come a time when your child thinks that you "just don't understand." If this happens, try to be realistic about what you can and can't do. If you find yourself unable to communicate with your child, you can try to find another person who can step in and fill that role. This might be a counselor at school, a younger relative, or even a sports coach. No one can be "all things" to their child, and you're no exception, regardless of your age. The important thing will be to make sure that your child gets the help he needs, whether it's from you or from someone else.

Loneliness

Most children of older parents, and especially those who were only children, expressed feeling great loneliness during their childhood. Part of the reason for this is that, when people postpone parenthood, family sizes are usually smaller. Not only do they tend to have only one child, but other relatives, such as cousins, uncles, and aunts, all tend to be older and aren't suitable companions for the child. Also, the child's grandparents, even if they are still alive, tend to be quite old and aren't able to participate actively in their grandchild's life. These feelings of loneliness can be overwhelming if both parents work, or if the parents don't actively participate in the child's activities.

Almost all of the adult children of older parents who were only children expressed regret at not having had a brother or sister, and of not having known their grandparents. As many expressed, there was no one with whom they could share their family history, and no one they could turn to for support, especially when their parents became old and ill.

Children of older single parents had a particularly tough time. Most had distasteful memories of their childhoods, and most linked their problems to the fact that they didn't have a father or any siblings. But, as Dr. Morris says in her study, there can be ways to fill the void. "Rather than sheltering the child from the outside world . . . or leaving him to struggle alone with his perceived inadequacies," she says, "parenting an only child seems to require a special perceptiveness, an even sharper awareness of needs than does parenting a child who is part of a larger family. On the one hand, it may require a willingness to let go, to share the child with others and allow the child exposure to the influence of those others. But the fine line between 'allowing the child exposure to the influence of others' and abandoning him or her may not always be clear to the child. . . . Children need to know they are loved and that they are important to their parents and that their parents will be available when they are needed. They need to feel protected—but not stifled."[7]

To help allay this feeling of loneliness, you could encourage your child to participate in activities that would help him broaden his circle of friends. This might be through the school, or by participating in church or community activities. Also, if you become active in school activities—for example, participating in the PTA—then your child would see you as a participant in *his* world, the world involving school and his friends. All of these things will help broaden your child's world and keep feelings of loneliness at bay.

Also, if your parents won't be alive, or will be quite old, by the time you have your child, you can search out substitute grandparents when the time is right. This might be through an older couple in your neighborhood, or a couple in a nearby nursing home. While these surrogate grandparents won't be able to regale the child with stories of you when you were his age, they can, if they so desire, supply the unconditional love and support of any grandparent.

Children need to be exposed to people of all ages. If your family circle isn't large, you can compensate by cultivating a broad social circle. It's through a broad circle of friends and relatives that a child can gain the feeling of belonging in the world.

Fear of Death

Another aspect of life that the children of older parents often have to face is death. Many of these children have an experience with death in the family at an early age, whether it's the death of a grandparent or the death of a parent. Also, many children of older parents, when they notice that their parents are older than the parents of their friends, fear that their parents will die. The feeling that their parents won't live to see them through college or into adulthood can become a haunting fear.

While you shouldn't raise the issue of death yourself, you'll want to be alert to any signs of worry. If your child begins to ask questions about your age or begins to say things like, "Mom, I wish you weren't so old so you wouldn't die soon," then address the issue. You'll be able to reassure the child by telling him that you're in good health, and that people live longer today than ever before.

Premature Role as Caretaker

And, finally, if you have children at a later age, you have to face the fact that your children may have to deal with your declining health while they're still relatively young. This is a prime situation in which resentment can build, especially when you consider that all of your children's friends will, at that time, be busy embarking on careers and living lives free from responsibility. The problem will be even worse if your child will be an only child; this means he'll be forced to shoulder the burden alone. As one child of an older parent said, "My father died when I was 28, and my mother is now in a nursing home with

Alzheimer's disease at the age of 75, while my friends' parents are enjoying their grandchildren."[8]

According to Robert Binstock, director of the Policy Center on Aging at the Heller School for Advanced Studies in Social Welfare, people have the greatest risk of contracting a disabling disease when they are around age 75.[9] If you have your children when you're in your early 40s, your child would only be in his early 30s when that occurs. And 32 is an awfully young age to have to assume care for a parent who has been debilitated by a stroke.

Once again, this is all the more reason to make sure that you take care of yourself. If you're planning on having children later in life, you need to be especially careful to ensure that your health will be at its best for as long as possible. This means exercising, eating a well-balanced, low-fat diet, and following your doctor's advice to the letter, when applicable. Furthermore, you should take pains to plan for your old age just as you plan for your child's college education. You should have a will, purchase necessary insurance policies, and set aside money for catastrophic illness. Your child may still feel the grief of losing a parent, or of having a parent who is ill, before his peers have even realized that life holds such possibilities. But, if you've planned carefully, he won't have to bear the burden of caring for you at a time when he should be focusing on his own life.

The Overall Assessment of Being an Older Parent

Probably nothing speaks louder than the actions of the adult children of older parents, and that action is that most of them have chosen to have their children before reaching age 30. According to those surveyed by Mr. Yarrow, 66% of all respondents, and 85% of those younger than age 30, said that their parents' ages influenced how they felt about when was the best time to have their children.[10] Some did say that having older parents exposed them to new possibilities, that delaying child-birth was an option, and that it might even be better to be older when having children. However, twice as many believed that it was better to have children earlier in life rather than later.

Some of their reasons for this belief were that they wanted to be healthy and active when their children became adults. They wanted to still be young enough to participate not only in their children's lives, but in their grandchildren's lives as well. They also stated that they wanted to have their children early enough so that they wouldn't become a burden to their children while their children were still young.

The Positive Aspects of Being Older

These adult children of older parents give anyone consider-ing having children later in life considerable food for thought. At the same time, though, let's keep everything in perspective. First of all, just because a child's parents are 26 years old when he's born doesn't mean that he's guaranteed to have healthy, active parents throughout his adult life. Even though they're relatively young, they could still die from a catastrophic illness, such as cancer or heart disease, or be killed in an accident. Life gives no guarantees.

Next, there are plenty of adult children of *younger* parents who can relate troubled childhoods. Don't forget that the major-ity of families in the United States today are dysfunctional. Chil-dren grow up dealing with divorce, alcoholism, child abuse, poverty, and a lack of love. Many, many factors influence a child's life. Only one of these is his parents' ages. For example, studies have shown that parents who are warm and nurturing tend to raise children who are independent and who are secure in their relations with others.[11] In contrast, the children of cool and inattentive parents tend to lack social skills.[12]

So, don't forget about all you have to offer. By postponing

parenthood until you're ready, you're guaranteeing that your child will be wanted and loved. By having taken care of your professional, financial, and emotional growth earlier, you'll be better prepared to devote the time necessary to raising well-balanced and happy children. Because you will have already experienced many of life's pleasures, you'll be more prepared to give them up to devote time to your child. In contrast, people who have children early in life haven't had the opportunity to develop their own identities, much less cultivate a strong bond with a spouse, before a newborn intrudes on their time and demands their attention. Sure, they may be able to play touch football with their child, but can they be as receptive to their child's needs as an older parent can? Are they as ready to sacrifice their own desires and personal satisfactions for the benefit of their child? If a parent is older, this requirement may be that much easier. By having lived longer, and experienced more, it becomes easier to make the trade-off.

Also, mothers who postpone parenthood tend to be better educated than do younger mothers, and this can pay off in benefits to the baby. For example, college-educated mothers tend to talk more to their babies. They also give their children more interesting toys to play with and they tend to use praise rather than criticism to teach their child.[13] They're also more patient with their children and, because they've been married longer, are much less likely to divorce.

Also, when considering your age, remember that people tend to stay healthier longer than they did a generation ago. Furthermore, as the population as a whole ages, by the time you become truly old and dependent, hopefully there will be more options for care than becoming dependent upon your children.

So, if you're older than the norm and planning on having children, you do need to be aware of these areas we discussed in which age can be a problem. But, if you truly want children, instead of letting these complaints discourage you, you should instead look upon them as guidelines as to how to structure your parenting. Older parents have a great deal to offer, especially if you take pains now to keep yourself in the best physical and mental shape possible. As Yale psychologist Edward Zigler said in a *Time* magazine article, "Good parenting is a process of bonding and attachment. This is more important than the age of the parent."[14]

5

Maintaining Your Fertility

To postpone parenthood, you must keep your reproductive organs in peak shape. You've already learned that aging affects your reproductive function; but that's not the only threat to your fertility. Everyday living exposes you to additional factors that can affect your chances for having a baby at some point in the future. While you can't control the fact that you're growing older, you can have some say as to whether environmental factors will take their toll on your reproductive abilities. Remember: the longer you live, and the more you're exposed to certain risk factors, the greater your chances are for developing infertility. Therefore, if you want to maximize your chances for having a baby later in life, you must act now to ensure your reproductive health. Below are some of the steps you should follow to keep your reproductive organs healthy and functioning.

Maintain a Mutually Monogamous Sexual Relationship

First and foremost, you need to limit yourself to one sexual partner, and, at the same time, you need to have confidence that your partner is doing the same. The reason for this is that sexually transmitted diseases, or STDs, cause about 20% of all cases of infertility in the United States.[1] What's especially tragic is that these diseases, and the resultant infertility, are *preventable*.

A woman's delicate reproductive organs are especially vulnerable to attack by STDs. To begin with, the bacteria that cause STDs latch onto sperm like parasites onto a whale. During intercourse, when the man ejaculates, the sperm and their disease-causing passengers are launched high into the woman's vagina. The sperm, in their eagerness to meet a ripe egg, scamper through the cervix and scatter throughout the uterus and fallopian tubes, sometimes even dropping out of the ends of the tubes into the peritoneal cavity. The sperm's widespread wandering suits the STD bacteria just fine; without any effort at all, the bacteria have invaded the sensitive and vulnerable territory of a woman's reproductive organs, where the normal secretions of the endometrium and fallopian tubes provide a perfect medium for bacterial spread. The bacteria move quickly throughout the reproductive organs, invading cells, secreting toxins, and causing painful inflammation. When the inflammation subsides, stiff and dysfunctional scar tissue is left in its place.

This generalized inflammation of the pelvic cavity is known as pelvic inflammatory disease, or PID. One of the worst things about this disease—besides the fact that it's capable of annihilating your reproductive organs—is that it can be difficult to diagnose. The key symptoms of PID are fever and abdominal pain; needless to say, these are the key symptoms of dozens of other illnesses as well, ranging from the flu to appendicitis. Many times, doctors don't diagnose PID until the symptoms become severe; by the time that happens, the reproductive organs may have been irreparably damaged. Sometimes the infection resolves on its own without ever having been treated. But you can be sure that the infecting organisms don't retreat without first scarring the pelvic cavity.

The main victims of an STD's scarring are the fallopian tubes. This is especially bad news as far as your future reproductive abilities are concerned. The fallopian tubes are extremely narrow; at their narrowest point, they are only 1/50 of an inch wide. As you can see, it doesn't take much scar tissue to completely occlude the tube. And if the tube is blocked, an egg can't descend and become fertilized. Even if the tube isn't completely blocked, problems can still result. Consider the fact that sperm are incredibly tiny, much smaller than the eggs you ovulate. This means that, even if your fallopian tube is blocked, sperm may be able to squirm past the blockage and meet and fertilize the egg on the other side. The sperm has accomplished its mission of fertilizing an egg; however, the egg is left in a terrible predicament. Once fertilized, it will begin to grow, despite the fact that it's stuck in the tight confines of the fallopian tube. This is what is known as an ectopic pregnancy. After just a short time of growth, the developing embryo will begin to strain against the sides of the fallopian tube, causing severe pain. Without treatment, the tube may rupture and hemorrhage. Even if this doesn't occur, treatment often involves surgically removing the fallopian tube.

Besides blocking the fallopian tubes, the scarring from PID serves yet another purpose. The nooks and crannies created by the scarred tissue are prime spots in which bacteria that arrive later can hide and launch new infections. This means that if you continue to expose yourself to infection, it will get easier and easier for harmful bacteria to create a raging case of PID. What's worse, each new infection will increase your risk for becoming infertile. Doctors estimate that just one bout of PID leaves a woman with a 15% chance of becoming infertile. After two infections, the chance increases to 50%, and, after three infections, her risk of infertility is as high as 75%.[2]

A variety of organisms can cause PID, almost all of which are sexually transmitted. Probably the most well-known organism is *Neisseria gonorrhoeae*, the cause of gonorrhea. Rampant throughout the world, more than 1 million cases of gonorrhea were reported in the United States in 1975, while experts estimate that more than 4 million cases went unreported. What's worse, experts also estimate that the number of cases increases by 15% each year.[3]

Between 10% and 17% of the women who contract gonorrhea develop an infection in their fallopian tubes.[4] This usually causes fever, abdominal pain, and a puslike vaginal discharge. Other women, though, may have few, or no, symptoms. In these instances, a woman is at the mercy of her partner to let her know that he was infected. And if she's not lucky enough to have had a partner who will own up to the truth, she could keep the infection lodged in her pelvis for some time before ever becoming aware of it. In the meantime, the bacteria would have exacted a toll on her reproductive organs.

Even more prevalent than gonorrhea, and perhaps more dangerous, is infection by *Chlamydia*. The *Chlamydia* is a tricky, unique organism, and not very well understood. It's not really a bacterium or a virus, but it invades cells the way a virus does. Once it gains entrance to a cell, *Chlamydia* multiplies inside the cell until the host cell can no longer maintain its boundaries. The cell then explodes, scattering the invading bacteria to other cells, which starts the process over again.

Chlamydia infections are potent. In fact, studies conducted in Sweden showed that just one attack of the *Chlamydia* parasite was three times more likely than gonorrhea to cause sterility in women. The danger of a *Chlamydia* infection is that it doesn't produce any symptoms, or, at best, produces very mild ones. This means that the organism can completely destroy a woman's reproductive organs without her ever knowing that she's infected. What's worse, the organism is very difficult to detect in culture, making it difficult to diagnose.

If you're sexually active with more than one partner, you may wish to request that you obtain a culture for *Chlamydia* as part of your routine checkup. But, if you ever have symptoms of low abdominal pain, a vaginal discharge, and a fever, and there's a possibility that you may have been exposed to *Chlamydia*, see your doctor immediately. If this is the case, the doctor should treat you as if you have the infection and prescribe a course of tetracycline for both you and your partner without waiting for the culture results. When dealing with an infection like *Chlamydia*, you don't have any time to waste.

Another mysterious bacterium that can cause problems is *Ureaplasma*. Not much is known about this organism, other than the fact that many infertile women seem to harbor the bacteria in their cervixes. Once treated with antibiotics, they often become pregnant. Researchers don't know why this is, but they do have a couple of theories. The first is that *Ureaplasma*, and a related strain called *Mycoplasma*, are part of the bacteria that normally live in the reproductive tracts of men and women, and that, for some unknown reason, the bacteria cause some women to be infertile. The second theory is that these bacteria somehow impair the body's ability to ward off other, more hostile bacteria, which then enter and cause PID.

Again, an infection by *Ureaplasma* or *Mycoplasma* causes no symptoms. Doctors usually only discover the infection when they're investigating another complaint. Once diagnosed, though, it can be treated with antibiotics.

Besides the risk you run of contracting a bacterial infection if you have sex with more than one partner, you also have a risk of picking up a viral infection. Sexually transmitted diseases caused by viruses include herpes simplex, venereal warts, and AIDS. Although viruses don't cause pelvic inflammation the way bacteria do, they can wreak their own kind of havoc with your reproductive system. For starters, they break down the protective cervical mucus, which allows hostile bacteria to enter and set up their own infections. Besides that, they disrupt the normal chemical environment of the vagina, making it inhospitable to sperm. But above all, remember that there are no cures for viruses. Once you contract a sexually transmitted virus, you'll have it forever. Then, when you decide to become pregnant, you'll have to deal with the possibility that you could pass the infection on to your infant. Or, in the case of AIDS, you'll have to worry whether you'll even survive long enough to raise your child.

To evaluate your risk for developing PID or contracting a viral infection, think about how many sexual partners you've had. If you became sexually active when you were a teenager, and you've had several different partners since you've been an adult, your risk is significant. Realize that the more partners you have, the more kinds of infecting agents you're exposing yourself to. The risk is only compounded if your partner also has had several different partners.

All in all, it's best to prevent these disorders by maintaining a mutually monogamous relationship. If that's not possible, just be very careful about with whom you have sex. Learn as much as you can about a potential partner's past sexual habits before you sleep with him. If he has had several different partners, then you may want to reconsider your choice. If you do decide to sleep with someone, further decrease your risk of contracting a sexually transmitted disease by always using a condom.

Furthermore, if you ever think that you may have been exposed to an infection, don't wait for symptoms to develop. Call your gynecologist immediately. Be specific about your concerns and ask for a test for gonorrhea or *Chlamydia*. Better yet, request that tests for these diseases be performed routinely as a part of your regular exam. Treated early, an STD doesn't have to result in PID. Likewise, if PID does occur, early treatment can keep fertility problems from resulting.

Use Appropriate Forms of Contraception

The next step in protecting your fertility is making sure that the type of contraception you use now to prevent becoming pregnant doesn't diminish your chances for giving birth in the future. The method of contraception that poses the greatest threat to women who have never had children is the intrauterine device (IUD).

Exactly how IUDs prevent pregnancy has never been clearly understood. They may block fertilization of the egg, or they may alter the lining of the uterus and prevent a fertilized egg from implanting. Regardless, doctors know that the IUD irritates the uterine lining. This irritation is more severe in women who have never had children because their uteruses are small. And, the more inflammation that exists, the more bacteria love it. This irritated tissue provides bacteria with an ideal location in which they can take hold and initiate an infection. And, as you know, an untreated infection can lead to PID.

Old-style IUDs were especially hazardous because the string that hung from the device acted as an entry way for disease-causing bacteria. Bacteria would breed in between the braided fibers of the string and then climb up into the uterus. Newer IUDs still have a string, but it's made of a single mono-filament fiber that resists bacteria. Such advances, and some recent studies, have led some to claim that the IUD may not be as risky as once thought.

However, most experts still feel that the IUD increases the user's risk for developing PID. Some experts claim that women who use IUDs have as much as a fourfold greater risk of developing PID than do women who use no contraceptives at all.[5] In addition, women with IUDs can develop low-grade infections of which they're not even aware but which scar their fallopian tubes just the same. This risk for infection is even greater if you have more than one sexual partner. Therefore, if having a baby in the future is very important to you, you would be better off having the IUD removed and using another form of contraception.

Perhaps the best contraceptives to use are barrier methods, such as the diaphragm or the condom. Besides being reliable (especially when used in conjunction with a spermicide), they don't change your body in any way. They simply block sperm that try to enter your uterus. In addition, this method of action may actually help protect your fertility. By keeping out sperm, these forms of contraception may help lower your risk for developing PID.

Some medical experts have also claimed that the birth control pill may help prevent PID. The reason for this is that birth control pills toughen the cervical mucus, which serves as sort of a shield against some disease-causing bacteria. One bacterium that isn't foiled by this change in mucus is *Chlamydia*. And since *Chlamydia* infection is the most prevalent STD today, there isn't much sense in depending on birth control pills to ward off STDs. Furthermore, using birth control pills over a long period of time can hamper your fertility in other ways.

To begin with, just because you stop taking the pill doesn't mean that ovulation will immediately restart. Most women don't begin menstruating until they've been off the pill for three or four months. For others, this lag time can be as long as a year. And if you've put off trying to become pregnant until late in your reproductive life, postponing for another year while you wait for your body to get back in sync could be intolerable, not to mention detrimental.

The reason this delay occurs is because of the way birth control pills work. The entire purpose of birth control pills is to block ovulation. It does this by substituting its own steady stream of hormones for your body's normal hormone pulsations. This causes your body to stop producing its own hormones and, when the hormones don't rise and fall as expected, your ovaries don't produce eggs. After awhile, your brain gets used to this infusion of hormones and forgets that it ever had to work for a living. When you suddenly stop taking birth control pills, it takes your brain awhile to comprehend that it has to produce again. As we've said before, this can take months. If the months begin to drag on, though, and your body still does not start producing hormones as it should, your doctor may prescribe a round of fertility drugs to jolt your body back to its senses.

Simply taking the pill for a long period of time doesn't seem to have any effect on how quickly your body returns to normal. However, other factors do seem to have an influence. One such factor is age; the lag time between stopping pills and resuming normal function is especially noticeable in older women. It's even worse, though, in women who started taking birth control pills when they were young, before their own menstrual patterns became regular. The same thing goes for women who were erratic in their use of the pill. Repeatedly going on and off the pill can confuse your body to the point that it takes months before resuming operation under its own hormonal power. Eventually, though, with or without help, most women resume normal ovulation and menstruation after discontinuing use of the pill.

If you're over age 30 and you're currently taking the pill,

and you know that you want to have children one day, it would probably be a good idea to stop taking the pill now. (Women who don't want children can usually safely take the pill until age 35, unless a medical condition dictates otherwise.) In the interim before you want to get pregnant, use a barrier method of contraception. Even if you want to become pregnant immediately, you should still wait three or four months after stopping the pill before trying to conceive. This way, your body has a chance to regain its own hormonal rhythm. If you get pregnant before you've restarted regular menstruation, it could be difficult to date exactly when the pregnancy began, which could be important later.

Don't Smoke

You may be tempted to skip this section, thinking that you already know that smoking is bad for you. Sure, you may be saying, smoking causes lung cancer and can harm the fetus if a woman smokes while pregnant. So let me tell you something you probably don't know: smoking now can interfere with your chances for becoming pregnant in the future.

For example, did you know that smokers tend to have earlier menopauses than do nonsmokers? It's true, with heavier smokers leading the way. Even light smokers tend to enter menopause earlier than do women who have never smoked. To illustrate, one study of 656 women found that the average age of menopause for women who had never smoked was 49.4 years. But, for women who smoked at least 15 cigarettes, or less than one pack, every day, the age at menopause was 47.6 years.[6] This is almost two years earlier than the women who never smoked. This becomes extremely significant when you consider, as was discussed earlier, that women become infertile as long as 10 years before menopause. So if you're planning to postpone childbearing until your late 30s, and you continue to smoke, then you could be setting yourself up for disappointment.

Why this accelerated menopause occurs isn't clear. One theory is that the nicotine found in cigarettes somehow influences the secretion of the hormones involved in the menopause process. Another theory is that smoking triggers the release of certain enzymes that alter the body's response to reproductive hormones.[7] Regardless of the cause, smoking cigarettes will decrease the amount of time you have available in which to reproduce.

Besides causing an accelerated menopause, smoking also seems to delay conception.[8] In fact, at least one study has shown that, if a woman smokes, her chances of becoming pregnant within one year are 25% less than the chances of a woman who doesn't smoke. And the risk increases with each cigarette smoked.

Researchers found in a separate study that women who smoked fewer than 20 cigarettes (or one pack) a day had a 25% reduction in fertility as compared to nonsmokers. At the same time, the fertility of women who smoked more than 20 cigarettes a day was cut nearly in half.[9] It isn't surprising then to learn that smokers report problems with infertility 46% more often than do nonsmokers.[10] In fact, doctors have discovered that women who have abnormalities in both their fallopian tubes and their cervixes are more likely to have been smokers. Smokers are also more likely to suffer ectopic pregnancies.[11]

Once again, researchers aren't absolutely certain why these problems occur. However, they do have some clues. For example, they know that cigarette smoke increases the force and amplitude of what are normally the gentle, wavelike movements of the fallopian tubes. Knowing this, they have theorized that this increase in tubal movements could interfere with fertilization and could also interfere with an egg's safe passage to the uterus.

But women aren't the only ones who need to be concerned about smoking affecting their fertility. Studies have shown that men who smoke have approximately 22% less sperm in an average semen sample as compared to men who don't smoke.[12] And it goes without saying that the fewer the number of sperm, the less the chances for fertilization.

But, even if you don't smoke, you're still not free from possible harm. Smoking is so pervasive in our society that it's impossible to avoid smoky environments altogether. Nevertheless, just being around people who smoke increases your risk for all of the ailments caused by smoking. Experts have estimated that smokers who work in a smoky environment inhale, through the secondhand smoke of others, the equivalent of one to three cigarettes a day. Even worse, the smoke that comes from the lighted end of a cigarette, and which makes up 80% of the smoke in a smoky room, contains higher concentrations of over 17 carcinogens than does exhaled smoke. Some experts have estimated that nonsmokers who remain in a very smoky room for one hour will inhale—just from the room smoke—a quantity of chemicals equivalent to that found in 10 to 15 cigarettes.[13]

Given all this evidence, there can be no other advice than "stop smoking." And if you don't smoke, avoid smoky environments as much as possible. If you work in an office with people who smoke, try to reposition your desk, or install a fan for ventilation, to minimize your exposure. You probably already know that smoking, and cigarette smoke, increase your risk for lung cancer, heart disease, and a variety of other ailments. If the threat of these diseases doesn't scare you, then remember that lighting up could influence your chances for having a child.

Evaluate Your Drinking Habits

The next life-style habit that you need to evaluate is how much you drink. It's well known that heavy drinking during pregnancy can result in fetal alcohol syndrome, a disorder that causes the infant to be born mentally retarded and with various deformities of the body and organs. But fetal abnormalities can occur at much lower levels of alcohol ingestion. Some studies have shown that women who drank just one or two drinks a day early in pregnancy tended to have children who had slow reaction times, short attention spans, and lower intelligence test scores.[14] Even a would-be father's drinking habits can affect the fetus.

One study found that the babies of fathers who regularly consumed two drinks a day, or five drinks at one sitting, weighed about 6.5 ounces less than did other babies. This held true regardless of whether the mother smoked or drank.[15] You also need to realize that having an infant who is small at birth means more than that the baby just needs to gain weight. It means that the baby is starting life underdeveloped, which is a definite handicap. The infant has an increased risk of dying shortly after birth, and, if he does survive, he runs a risk of having a learning disability later in life.

Furthermore, if a man abuses alcohol, his sperm production often declines and, if that's not enough, the sperm that are produced may be less potent.[16] The reason for this is that alcohol, over time, damages the liver. One of the main functions of the liver is to clear used hormones from the body. If the liver is damaged from alcohol use, it can't perform this function efficiently. As a result, female hormones—normally present in small amounts—begin to accumulate. In turn, this interferes with sperm production. And finally, extreme alcohol abuse can cause a man to be impotent.

As far as you're concerned, even though you may not be trying to get pregnant at this point, it is still worthwhile to evaluate your drinking habits. No one knows how much, if at all, alcohol affects the eggs that you currently have. But why take the risk? Also, keep in mind that, once you do conceive, the embryo will be alive and growing for at least two weeks before you even know you're pregnant. This means that anything you ingest during those early weeks could affect the developing embryo and could even influence whether the embryo implants.

If you currently drink, the best course is simply to cut back during your years of postponement. Besides minimizing the other harmful effects of alcohol, you can be assured that the eggs you have won't be harmed by the alcohol you ingest while waiting to conceive. Then, once you start trying to conceive, keep a handle on what, and how much, you consume. After years of postponement, and perhaps with a short time available in which to conceive, you wouldn't want to risk harming your child with excess alcohol consumption.

Avoid Using Recreational Drugs

Just as with alcohol, there's no question that, once you're pregnant, you should not take any type of drug—recreational, prescription, or over-the-counter—without first talking with your doctor. But, what about the years before conception?

Unfortunately, there is no hard-and-fast evidence about the effect that drugs have on your reproductive potential. However, it stands to reason that, because you already have all of the eggs you're ever going to have, it would be best to avoid all drug use. This becomes especially significant when you consider that some drugs, such as marijuana, can stay in the body for days or weeks, and perhaps even months. Also, because marijuana interferes with the production of testosterone, men who smoke may have a decreased sperm count.

Avoid Environmental Toxins

The next thing that can affect your future fertility are environmental toxins. We live in a world that is filled with chemicals. Some of these chemicals are known to cause cancer or birth defects. With others, it's more uncertain. While it would be impossible to try to cover this topic in any depth here, it's worth calling your attention to the fact that your environment at work and at home may contain chemicals that could affect your ability to give birth to a healthy child.

Your first requirement is simply to become aware of the chemicals to which you are exposed at work and at home. These may be chemicals that you touch, ingest, or even inhale. After that, you should take precautions to minimize your exposure to the chemicals. For example, if you work as a hairdresser, wear gloves when you apply dyes or hair permanent solutions. If your hobby is refinishing furniture, make sure that you work in a well-ventilated room.

Also, don't write off the chemicals that your partner might be exposed to as inconsequential. Substances that are common in certain occupations—such as lead, boron, cadmium, manganese, mercury, organic compounds, and pesticides—can cause a man's sperm to become abnormal, which increases the risk for birth defects and can also increase a woman's risk for miscarriage. Some of these same substances can also cause a reduction in sperm counts. Furthermore, lead and the pesticide DBCP (dibromochloropropane) can cause infertility. People who are at risk for being exposed to lead in the workplace include painters, battery workers, smelters, and artists.

Along the same line, if you or your partner work around X-rays, you need to make sure that you protect your genital areas with an appropriate radiation shield. X-rays not only interfere with the production of sperm, but they can also damage the sperm themselves; this can render the sperm incapable of fertilizing an egg or, if they can fertilize an egg, cause them to create birth defects. Even cells that produce sperm can be damaged, sometimes permanently.

If you have serious concerns about chemicals to which you may be exposed, contact the National Institute for Occupational Safety and Health or the Environmental Protection Agency for more information. On a state level, you might want to contact your state's public health or environmental regulation division for information on specific chemicals.

The point is not to trust blindly that everything in your environment is safe, because it's not. Try to learn about those chemicals in your environment that are dangerous, and then eliminate, or at least minimize, your exposure. And while you should be scrupulous in your attempt to minimize your exposure to chemicals and toxins, don't become obsessed. Keep in mind that, despite all of these toxins in our environment, most babies are born normal.

Maintain Appropriate Levels of Exercise

Pregnancy is physically demanding, no matter what a woman's age. But women over age 35 are more likely to feel the physical strains of pregnancy. By this stage of life, a person's body isn't used to growing and changing; for years, it's been in a steady state of maintenance. Pregnancy alters all that because it causes a woman's body to grow and change daily. If that's not enough, the extra weight of pregnancy stresses joints and muscles that already have experienced years of wear and tear.

You can prepare for these physical demands by making sure that you're in top physical shape before you conceive. You should maintain your physical assets throughout your years of pregnancy postponement by regularly engaging in aerobic exercise. Possibilities include bicycling, swimming, or fast walking. It's also a good idea to perform specific exercises to strengthen your lower back and abdominal muscles. These are the muscles that are forced to carry the lion's share of extra pregnancy weight, and you'll want to keep them toned and strong.

Although you want to make sure that you're physically ready for the demands of pregnancy, don't overdo your exercise regimen. While too little exercise may be harmful, so is too much. Studies show that excessive exercise can disrupt ovulation, often without the women even being aware that there's a problem. Also, once you become pregnant, exercising strenuously enough to raise your core body temperature to 102° F during the early weeks of pregnancy can damage the organs of the developing embryo, or can even trigger a miscarriage.

This can occur more easily than you might think, especially when you consider that a woman's body temperature normally climbs a half a degree with pregnancy. Also, if you exercise when it's hot or humid, your body can't dissipate heat quickly.

As a result, your core body temperature can reach a dangerous level before you know it.

In summary, make an effort to keep your muscles, your lungs, and your heart in good shape for the physical demands of a delayed pregnancy. If you tend to exercise strenuously, slack off just slightly on the intensity and length of your workouts once you begin trying to conceive. This way, you can still exercise enough to enjoy the physical benefits of exercise without worrying about affecting your fertility or harming a developing embryo.

Eat a Balanced Diet

Along the same line as getting an adequate amount of exercise, eating a balanced diet will help ensure that your body is ready for a pregnancy when the time is right. This means consuming the right proportions of carbohydrates, proteins, and fats as well as an adequate supply of vitamins. If you're not sure whether your diet is balanced, consult a nutritionist. It will be money well spent. Not only will it pay off in keeping you healthy now, it will help ensure that your infant will be healthy when you do choose to conceive.

To illustrate how what you eat before you conceive can affect your infant, consider a study of women in northern England, Scotland, Wales, and Ireland. This study found that women who took multivitamins containing folic acid (one of the B vitamins) for 28 days before conceiving, and then up until their second missed menstrual period, had a much smaller risk for having a baby with a neural tube defect.[17] You may recall that neural tube defects include spina bifida, which is an incomplete closure of the spinal column, and anencephaly, which is an incomplete development of the brain and skull. This study has been criticized by some as not being conclusive, so don't bank on it as being absolute. However, it does make a point that the quality of your diet before you conceive can affect the health of your infant. Besides that, although no one knows for sure, the quality of your diet now just might help preserve the integrity of your eggs for that extra length of time you need. There is no scientific basis for this, but why not maximize your chances as best you can?

At any rate, good nutrition and vitamin intake can't hurt, just as long as you don't overdo it with excessive vitamin supplements. While an adequate vitamin intake is important for a healthy fetus, vitamin overdoses, such as from megavitamin therapy, can cause birth defects.

Along with consuming an adequate supply of vitamins and nutrients, it's also important to keep an eye on the amount of calories you consume. If you weigh more than 20% over your ideal body weight, you should lose weight before trying to conceive. To begin with, overweight women tend to have ovulatory disorders. The reason for this is that fat cells play a role in secreting estrogen. As you know, your body needs hormones to peak and plummet in a cycle in order to ovulate. When excess fat cells are present, they dampen the hormonal peaks produced by the ovaries by releasing a steady stream of estrogen. As a result, ovulation may be impaired.

Besides ovulatory disorders, obese women are also at risk for a host of problems during pregnancy, including diabetes and high blood pressure. Also, overweight women tend to have large babies, which could make delivery complicated or necessitate the use of forceps or even a cesarean section. Furthermore, once you become pregnant, you won't be able to diet because you'll need to be concentrating on providing your growing infant with all of the nutrients it needs. All in all, it's safer for you—before, during, and after your pregnancy—to lose all excess weight before trying to conceive.

At the same time, if you weigh less than you should, you need to make a serious effort to gain weight. It's a well-known fact that underweight women have a greater incidence of infertility than do women who are of ideal weight. Some experts believe than being as little as 5% below your ideal body weight can hamper your chances for becoming pregnant. The reason for this is that, when you're underweight, you have a reduced amount of body fat; this, in turn, reflects a decreased amount of estrogen storage and production. And, as you already know, estrogen is one of the key reproductive hormones.

Dr. G. William Bates, the Director of Reproductive Endocrinology at South Carolina's Greenville Hospital System, feels that upping your weight by just 5% will significantly improve estrogen storage and production.[18] His rationale for this is that a 5% gain in weight results in a 15% increase in body fat.

To find your ideal weight, consult the height and weight table published by the Metropolitan Life Insurance Company. You can obtain a copy of this chart by sending a self-addressed, stamped envelope to Health and Safety Education, MetLife Insurance Company, 1 Madison Avenue, New York, NY 10010. When you consult the chart, keep in mind that the figures are calculated to include 3 pounds of clothes and 1-inch heels.

One final note about diet concerns caffeine. A study conducted a few years back raised a lot of interest when it concluded that consuming caffeinated beverages might cause some women to have difficulty conceiving. However, larger studies performed since that date have not made such a correlation. Researchers from the Centers for Disease Control and Harvard Medical School questioned 2817 women who had recently given birth about their consumption of coffee, decaffeinated coffee, tea, and colas. When they tabulated the results, there was no correlation between delayed conception and caffeine consumption of up to 7000 mg/month (which translates into a little more than two cups of drip coffee a day).[19]

In conclusion, take a good look at your diet now, before you ever try to conceive, and see to it that you consume an adequate amount of nutrients and the recommended number of calories. Not only will it help you be healthier now, it will promote the health of your long-awaited-for infant.

Obtain a Gynecological Evaluation

As soon as you start thinking about postponing parent-hood, you should make an appointment with your gynecologist to discuss the matter. What you learn here could strongly influ-ence when you decide to try to become pregnant. If you learn that you have a problem that may make it difficult for you to conceive or to carry to term, you most likely won't want to postpone your attempts at conception until the last possible minute. Also, if you learn that you have a disorder that could affect your fertility, but that it can be treated, you may choose to go ahead and take care of the problem ahead of time. Below are some guidelines as to how to structure your prepregnancy meet-ing with your doctor, and some of the information you should learn in this discussion.

Discussion of Medical History

First, be specific about the information you're seeking. Tell your doctor that you're planning to postpone pregnancy and that you want to know the risks you may face. Ask how any medical problems you currently have—such as diabetes, cardiac disease, high blood pressure, thyroid problems, or any other disorder—might influence your ability to conceive. Also, if you take any prescription or over-the-counter drugs on a regular basis, ask whether these would have any effect on your fertility or on the fetus once you conceive. When discussing your history with the doctor, be sure to mention any surgery that you've had in the past, and ask whether that surgery could have any effect on your ability to reproduce. This is particularly pertinent if you've ever had abdominal surgery, which can cause scar tissue and adhesions to develop in the pelvic cavity. In turn, these adhesions can lead to infertility. The doctor will also want to know if you've ever had a ruptured appendix or a ruptured ovarian cyst, conditions that can also cause scar tissue to form.

Evaluation of Risk for Genetic Abnormalities

After you've discussed your medical history and the current state of your health, you'll want to explore whether you are at risk for having a child with a genetic disorder. This is different from your risk for having a child with a chromosomal abnormality, such as Down's syndrome, which we discussed earlier. Those abnormalities are due to aging. The genetic risks we're talking about here are specific abnormalities in your chromosomes that you may be predisposed to because of your ethnic background or family history.

At this meeting, the doctor may ask you whether certain disorders have appeared in any members of your or your husband's family. If so, this could be a clue that you are at risk for passing these particular abnormalities along to your child. Some disorders seem to occur primarily in certain ethnic groups. For example, people of eastern European or Ashkenazic Jewish descent may be unknowing carriers of Tay–Sachs disease, a terrible disease in which the child deteriorates mentally and physically until he dies, usually by age three. Blacks risk passing along sickle cell anemia to their children, while people of Greek or Italian heritage risk having a child with thalassemia, which, in some forms, is a severe, incurable anemia.

Before you visit the doctor, think hard about your family background and have your partner do the same. Do you remember anyone having diseases such as muscular dystrophy; cystic fibrosis; Down's syndrome; bleeding disorders; spina bifida; heart, kidney, or liver ailments; or limb deformities? It might be easier to try to remember anyone who had a child who was particularly ill, who had unusual features, who died very young, or who was mentally slow. If you remember anything unusual about your family history—or if your spouse does about his—then mention it to your doctor. It's possible that a referral for genetic counseling is in order.

A genetic counselor is trained to gather the specific medical facts that apply to you. He, or she, will then analyze those facts and translate the information into risk factors. If indicated, you can undergo chromosome testing to see if you carry certain abnormal genes. Once you have this information, you can decide how to proceed with your plans for parenthood: whether you are willing to take the risk of conceiving a handicapped child, or whether you wish to pursue other options, such as adoption. Remember, though, that no preconception test can identify every possible genetic abnormality. In normal populations, there is still about a 3% chance of having a child with some type of genetic disorder.

Physical Examination

Next, you'll want to have a thorough physical exam, including a Pap smear and a mammogram, if indicated. Then, each year thereafter, it's important to continue to have these basic health evaluations. If any type of abnormality develops during your years of postponement—such as a lump in your breast or cervical cancer—then it can be diagnosed early and treated before you conceive. If you don't have these annual examinations, and the doctor discovers an abnormality that requires surgery after you're already pregnant, then the well-being of the fetus could be in jeopardy. Having surgery during the first three months of pregnancy increases the risk for having a miscarriage. You could also be faced with making a decision between receiving treatment, such as chemotherapy or radiation therapy, which could harm the fetus you may have waited years to conceive, or delaying treatment, which could endanger your life and health.

All in all, it's best to monitor your health closely so that you can recognize, and resolve, any health problems as soon as they develop. That way, you'll never be in the predicament of having to choose between your health and that of your unborn child.

Screening for Infections

This pregnancy postponement visit is a good time to receive blood tests to make sure you're immune to certain infections that could affect the fetus once you become pregnant. The first infection to test for is rubella (German measles). The rubella virus is particularly troublesome because, if contracted during the first eight weeks of pregnancy, there would be an extremely high chance that your baby would be born blind, deaf, or mentally retarded. The good news is that if you've had a full-blown case of German measles in the past, or if you've received an immunization, then your body would have produced antibodies to the virus and you won't be in danger of passing the infection on to your baby. To determine whether or not you're immune only requires a simple blood test. If the blood test shows that you have an adequate supply of rubella antibodies, then you can rest easy that you're immune to the virus. If you're not immune, this is the perfect time to receive a vaccination. After receiving the vaccination, you need to wait at lease three months before becoming pregnant to make sure that you don't pass the virus on to your child. But, once you've received the vaccine, you will be immune to rubella for life.

Another infection for which you may wish to be screened is toxoplasmosis. *Toxoplasma* is a parasite, often passed through raw or undercooked meat or cat litter. In adults, the infection usually only produces mild, flulike symptoms; however, if contracted during pregnancy, the illness can cause your infant to be born with serious birth defects. The problem with waiting until you're pregnant to be tested for toxoplasmosis is that a single, positive test result can't distinguish between a recent infection (one that could harm the fetus) and one that occurred in the past and no longer poses a threat. Think about that for a minute: you're pregnant, and you've just been informed that you have a positive test result for toxoplasmosis. But, the nurse tells you, they can't tell you whether you contracted the infection while you were pregnant—meaning that your child could be affected—or whether you contracted the infection years before, in which case the child wouldn't be affected at all. Imagine the months of anxiety you would have to endure, not knowing whether or not you were carrying a normal child. To avoid that anxiety, you should have the screening now, before you want to conceive. This way, if the test is positive, you'll know that you'll be immune to the illness once you decide to try to become pregnant. And, if it's negative, the doctor will at least have the opportunity to discuss with you how to avoid contracting such an infection.

A third blood test that you may also wish to have run is the test for the hepatitis B virus. The hepatitis B virus can remain dormant in some individuals, without their ever knowing they have the infection. If that's true in your case, and you become pregnant, there is a 70 to 90% chance that you'll pass the virus along to your infant. If you do, and the infant doesn't receive an immediate vaccination after birth, then he has an increased risk for developing severe liver disease after he becomes an adult. The individuals who are most at risk for contracting hepatitis B are health care workers who have contact with blood. If you work in such a field, you should seriously consider being vaccinated against the virus before you try to conceive.

The last blood test you may wish to receive is one to check your blood for abnormal blood antibodies. These antibodies develop in women with Rh-negative blood who have been exposed to Rh-positive blood cells. This can occur during an abortion, a miscarriage, a cesarean section, or, although infrequent, a mismatched blood transfusion. If you have developed such antibodies, and you conceive another child who also has Rh-positive blood, then that infant is at risk for erythroblastosis fetalis, a grave blood disorder that can lead to the infant's death. Therefore, if you have Rh-negative blood, and you've ever been in one of these situations where you may have been exposed to foreign blood cells, then you need to have your blood tested. Knowing this ahead of time could help in your quest for a healthy child.

Evaluation of Risks for Infertility

The last thing you'll want to do at this visit is ask the doctor to evaluate you, as best he can, for any disorders that could increase your risk for being infertile once you decide to try to conceive. This is extremely important to do now, before you even want to become pregnant. Too many women postpone childbearing until their houses, careers, and bank accounts are in order, only to learn that a particular disorder is blocking their ability to get pregnant—a disorder that could have been recognized, treated, and possibly resolved, if only they had started earlier. Remember that treatment for infertility takes time. And, if you postpone childbearing until late in your reproductive life, you won't have any time to waste, especially not on treatments that could have been completed years earlier. Following are some of the disorders that could affect the future fertility of you or of your partner. Being attentive to this aspect of your health now will help you recognize potential problems *before* you begin counting down the days to conception. This extra cushion of time will then allow you either to take steps to resolve the problem, or at least to adjust your plans for pregnancy accordingly.

Endometriosis

Endometriosis is called the "career woman's disease" because it often strikes women over age 30 who have never been pregnant. Affecting between four and ten million women, endometriosis results when endometrial tissue occurs in places other than where it belongs, which is inside the uterus. You may recall that endometrial tissue normally lines the inside of the uterus; each month, it swells with blood as it waits for a fertilized egg. If no fertilized egg arrives, the endometrium sloughs off, resulting in menstruation.

In endometriosis, bits of endometrial tissue crop up on the ovaries, the fallopian tubes, the floor of the pelvic cavity, the outer surface of the uterus, the bowel, or on other organs inside the pelvis. Exactly how the endometrial tissue ends up existing outside the uterine cavity isn't clear. Experts know that, during menstruation, some of the menstrual flow, instead of exiting the body through the vagina like it should, backs up into the fallopian tubes and spills out into the pelvic cavity. The tissues in the pelvic cavity usually absorb this misdirected flow without any problem. However, the experts suspect that, in some women, for reasons they don't understand, this misdirected flow plants itself on various organs. Once it has taken up residence, it begins its own monthly ritual of swelling and shedding.

Another theory is that endometriosis actually develops *in utero*, when the reproductive organs are first being formed. According to this explanation, some of the cells meant to line the uterine cavity get lost and end up in other locations. These cells may lie dormant for years, but once puberty strikes, the cells begin to grow. Other investigators feel that there may be some genetic link for the disease, because endometriosis tends to crop up among different members of the same family.

Each month, when the female hormones rise and fall in their normal cycle, this misplaced tissue reacts just like the endometrium: it swells and, when menstruation occurs, it bleeds. But this blood can't exit the body like normal endometrial tissue can. Instead, it's forced to flow onto the organs on which the endometrial tissue resides. This irritates the delicate tissue of the organs; inflammation results and the areas become red, swollen, and painful. Eventually, some of these patches of errant tissue burst, scattering tiny seeds of endometrial tissue onto other organs. And so the disease spreads. This pattern repeats itself month after month, and the constant irritation caused by the swelling and bleeding triggers the formation of scar tissue. These scars, when severe, can encase the reproductive organs: they can block the fallopian tubes, interfere with ovulation, and bind the fallopian tube as it reaches for an ovulating egg. In addition, endometriosis may change the quality of the fluid that normally coats your pelvic cavity, making it toxic to sperm; it may also disrupt the production of key female hormones. It is not entirely clear whether small amounts of endometriosis interfere with fertility, but it is clear that large amounts of the errant tissue can irreparably damage a woman's reproductive organs. And if that's not bad enough, endometriosis *may* increase the risk for having a miscarriage. Some researchers have cited evidence that women with untreated endometriosis have a miscarriage rate ranging from 20 to 70%.[20] However, other researchers have questioned these findings and feel that the miscarriage rate in women with endometriosis may not be that high, after all.[21]

Perhaps the most important aspect of endometriosis that you should consider is that, the more cycles that this renegade tissue is allowed to swell and bleed, the more scar tissue that is likely to result. That's why this disease is so risky for women who want to postpone parenthood. Pregnancy, you see, at least gives the tissue of your abdominal cavity a nine-month respite from the swelling and bleeding of endometriosis. One or two of these breaks at an early age help to lessen the damage from this disease. But without this reprieve, the damage can be severe by the time a busy career woman decides she wants to become pregnant.

So, you're saying, how can I know in advance if I have endometriosis? Unfortunately, knowing for certain that you have endometriosis, or even how severe it is, isn't that easy. Certain symptoms may give you a clue. One of the most common symptoms is pain before and during menstruation. Now, before you get too excited, realize that this isn't a definitive symptom. Many woman who *don't* have endometriosis have menstrual cramps. To focus in a little more on whether the pain that may accompany your period is related to endometriosis, consider these questions: Did your menstrual cramps start later in life, after several years of menstruation with no cramping?

Or, if you've always had cramps, have they worsened in severity over the past several years? Do you have back pain with your period? Does it hurt to have a bowel movement about the time of menstruation? Do you feel pain during intercourse with deep penetration? If you answered "yes" to any of these questions, then the pain you feel every month *may* be related to endometriosis. And even if you do have pain that sounds like it may be related to endometriosis, and the pain is severe, that doesn't necessarily mean that your endometriosis is severe.

Some women who suffer severe pain actually have very mild endometriosis; on the other hand, some women have no pain but actually have extensive disease.

After pain, one of the most common symptoms—and sometimes the only symptom—is infertility. In fact, endometriosis is responsible for 25 to 30% of all cases of infertility in women.[22] For women who have postponed childbearing, infertility as the only symptom is especially distressing. By the time she finds out she has endometriosis, there might not be enough time left on her biological clock to effectively treat the disease.

Another symptom that could give you a clue that something might be wrong is a change in your menstrual pattern. Some women with endometriosis find that their flow becomes heavy or prolonged, that their cycle changes in frequency, or that they have unexplained spotting or bleeding between periods.

During your physical exam, your doctor might be able to feel some endometrial growths. However, he won't be able to tell how extensive the endometriosis is, or even where the growths are located. The only way to know for sure whether or not you have endometriosis, or how severe it is, is to undergo a surgical procedure called a laparoscopy. To have the procedure performed, you would be admitted to the hospital on an outpatient basis and placed under general anesthesia. The doctor would then make a tiny incision in your abdomen and insert a fiber-optic tube called a laparoscope. The doctor would then look through the tube and scan the organs inside your abdominal cavity in an effort to locate any pesky outgrowths of endometrial tissue.

Of course, at this stage, when you're not even sure when you're going to have children, you probably don't want to subject yourself to such a procedure. However, if you have any of the classic symptoms of endometriosis—such as the characteristic pain or a family history of the disease—then you might want to consider having an evaluation now. That way, if you do have endometriosis, you could decide on a course of treatment that could make the difference in whether or not you'll be able to have children when you're ready. Also, if you're over age 35, and you find that you're still not pregnant after six months of trying, you would be wise to get a medical evaluation. You would hate not to discover that endometriosis was blocking your chances for conception until it was too late for treatment to have much of an effect.

But knowing for certain that you have endometriosis isn't the only problem. Deciding how to treat it is an entirely different conundrum. To begin with, there is no cure for this rather relentless disease. Treatment simply strives to decrease the symptoms and enhance fertility by eradicating as much of the actively bleeding tissue as possible. To further complicate matters, the best route for reaching this goal is the subject of controversy.

Oftentimes, when the endometriosis is mild and produces few symptoms, doctors recommend simply observing the condition for awhile. Some women may find, after a period of time, that the condition has resolved on its own, or that they were able to conceive without too much difficulty. But, if the condition worsens, the doctor would probably want to institute a course of drug therapy. And, depending upon your age and how long you want to wait before having children, he may recommend that you try drug therapy right from the start.

At one time, doctors prescribed birth control pills in a dosage high enough to stop menstruation altogether. This created a sort of "pseudopregnancy" during which the endometrial tissue wouldn't swell and bleed and would stop causing further damage. This is still the best route for some younger women with endometriosis who want to check the disease until they are ready to get pregnant. Of course, for older women, there are the other problems of birth control pills to consider, such as a delayed return of ovulation. This would be one option to discuss with your doctor, though, if you feel you are at risk for having endometriosis but want to delay childbearing.

For symptomatic endometriosis, the most commonly prescribed drug is danazol. Danazol is a synthetic male hormone that suppresses the production of estrogen and, along with it, ovulation. In effect, the drug creates a state of pseudo-menopause. Again, since the endometriosis is deprived of the monthly surges of estrogen it needs to swell, it begins to shrink. But there are disadvantages to this treatment, the first of which is that it takes months to achieve results. And, if you've waited until the last possible minute to try to conceive, this could be the death knell for your plans for pregnancy. The other disadvantage is that at least half of the women who take the drug experience undesirable side effects. These include weight gain, acne, decreased breast size, the growth of excessive body and facial hair, hot flashes, mood changes, and excessive sweating. Less frequently, some women experience a permanent deepening of their voice.

Another concern about taking danazol is that it lowers the level of high-density lipoprotein (HDL) in the blood; HDL is what is known as the "good" cholesterol. Researchers have found that a woman's blood cholesterol returns to normal after she's been off the drug for three to five months. However, doctors feel that even this temporary drop in HDL may increase the risk for developing atherosclerosis and heart disease at some later date. For this reason, doctors advise against taking the drug for longer than about six months.[23]

Finally, even though the goal of danazol therapy is to stop ovulation, you may still ovulate in the beginning of therapy when dosages are low. Because this medication could harm the fetus if you were to conceive, you would need to use a barrier method of contraception while taking the drug.

If those aren't enough disadvantages to danazol therapy, consider its expense. The usual six- to nine-month course of 400 mg (two tablets) twice a day may cost more than $1400. Furthermore, the six to nine months you're taking danazol are six to nine months you'd be forced to postpone trying to conceive. All the more reason to try to identify this problem as early as possible.

Once you finish a course of danazol, it's uncertain how much, or even whether, your chances for pregnancy will be improved. Exact pregnancy rates are less than clear because some studies that report an increased pregnancy rate didn't differentiate between women who had mild or severe disease, while others used varying doses of medication. Overall, though, some experts have reported pregnancy rates after danazol treatment ranging from 28 to 72%.[24]

Remember, though, danazol does not cure endometriosis; it merely arrests it. Once you stop taking the medication, the disease can return. In fact, between 6 and 12 months after the medication is stopped, the disease, and its symptoms, return in over one-third of the cases. This means that if you begin taking danazol, you should be prepared to begin trying to conceive as soon as you stop the therapy.

You may be thinking that, even if you only have mild endometriosis, you may want to take the drug during your time of postponement just to buy yourself a little more time. However, it doesn't seem to work that way. Even women with mild endometriosis who have had difficulty conceiving haven't seemed to benefit from danazol. For example, a study compared a group of women with mild endometriosis who took danazol to a group of women with mild endometriosis who received no treatment. After six months of observation, only 6, or 30%, of the 20 women who took danazol became pregnant. On the other hand, 14, or 50%, of the 28 women who received no treatment conceived. After one year, the results were similar: more of the women who had received no treatment were pregnant as opposed to the women who had received treatment.[25] This would naturally lead someone to question whether it would be appropriate to take danazol for mild endometriosis if the only purpose is to enhance fertility.

Besides danazol, there is another medication used to treat endometriosis. This medication, which is fairly new on the scene, is synthetic gonadotropin-releasing hormone (GnRH). Under normal conditions, the pituitary gland in the brain secretes GnRH in a pulsatile fashion. This series of hormone bursts stimulates the release of follicle-stimulating hormone

(FSH) and luteinizing hormone (LH). As discussed in Chapter 1, these two hormones are essential if the ovary is to release mature eggs. But, researchers have discovered that, if they give synthetic GnRH in a steady, continuous dose, the ovaries are turned off by the hormone's persistence and shut down production. As a result, the level of estrogen drops. Without estrogen to stimulate its monthly cycle, the endometriosis shrinks.

Administered through injections and intranasal spray over a seven- to eight-month period, synthetic GnRH has shown promising results in the treatment of endometriosis. In addition, the side effects with synthetic GnRH therapy are less severe than with danazol; the most common side effects are hot flashes and vaginal dryness, which are simply related to the low levels of estrogen. Doctors have found, too, that if they prescribe a progesterone supplement along with the medication, the symptoms become much less noticeable.

The last treatment for endometriosis is surgery. This may be recommended if medication therapy doesn't work, if the endometriosis is particularly severe, or if you've discovered the disease late in your reproductive life when you don't have the time medication needs to work. To treat endometriosis surgically, your doctor would most likely use a laparoscope (just like was used to diagnose the disorder) to see inside your peritoneal cavity. Then, once he spots the areas of endometriosis, he can destroy the lesions by burning them with electrical coagulation, cutting them out with a knife, or, as is most common today, "evaporating" them with a laser.

Surgical treatment seems to be especially successful in women who have severe disease. Pregnancy success rates after surgery range from 30 to 75%, depending upon the severity of the disease.[26] If you ever feel that you are a candidate for this type of surgery, it is extremely important that you seek out a doctor who has extensive experience using the laser to treat endometriosis. Remember that your fallopian tubes are very fragile; you wouldn't want anyone with less than expert hands aiming the laser.

DES Exposure

DES, or diethylstilbestrol, is a synthetic estrogen that was given to many pregnant women during the 1950s to reduce the risk of miscarriage. It has become apparent through the years that the daughters of women who took DES have an increased risk for vaginal cancer and also have a propensity to develop endometriosis. Furthermore, these same women tend to have uterine deformities; particularly, the uterus is shaped like the letter "T" instead of its normal upside-down pear shape. This T-shaped uterus doesn't expand well during pregnancy and, therefore, the women have an increased risk for premature delivery and miscarriage. Another problem that occurs in women who were exposed to DES *in utero* is that they may have a weak, or incompetent cervix. When the weight of a developing fetus increases beyond a certain point, usually well before the required nine months have expired, the cervix gives way and a miscarriage or premature birth results.

If you know for a fact that your mother took DES when she was pregnant with you, you may want to be evaluated sooner than you had planned so that you can determine whether you have a T-shaped uterus. In the meantime, though, don't despair that you'll never be able to have children. Some statistics show that 60% of DES daughters are able to carry a pregnancy to term. Only 20% never conceive, and another 20% have repeated miscarriages.[27]

If you're not sure whether or not your mother took DES, try to find out. Your mother would have been a candidate for taking the drug if she has ever had a miscarriage before becoming pregnant with you, or if she has had any abnormal bleeding during her pregnancy. To know for certain whether or not you were exposed, you may need to do a little detective work.

First, if possible, ask your mother if she remembers taking anything while she was pregnant with you. If your mother is deceased, you could try to track down her obstetrician; his name would be on your birth certificate. Some doctors, although retired, keep all of their records and would be able to look up the information for you. If you have no luck there, your best bet would simply be an examination by your doctor. A woman who was exposed to DES *in utero* tends to have a slightly misshapen vagina or cervix. Next, a doctor can also perform an outpatient X-ray test to determine whether you have a T-shaped uterus. (This test is discussed in detail in Chapter 8.)

If you do find out for certain that you were exposed to DES *in utero*, you'll want to take that into consideration when planning when to try to become pregnant. Simply realizing that you may have difficulty carrying a child to term could mean that you want to get a jump on trying to conceive.

Uterine Fibroids

Fibroid tumors are benign growths inside the muscle of the uterus. The older you get, the more prone you are to developing one or more of these growths. In fact, one out of every four women between the ages of 30 and 50 have uterine fibroids.[28] Many times, your doctor can feel fibroid tumors when he performs a physical exam. He may also use an ultrasound to locate the fibroids and to learn how large they are.

Most of the time you won't have any symptoms of these growths and they won't present any problems. If they do cause symptoms, the most common complaints include heavy menstrual flow, irregular bleeding, backache, and abdominal pain. Even without these symptoms, though, fibroid tumors may interfere with your ability to have a child. Depending upon the location, the tumor may keep the embryo from implanting properly. This is especially true if the fibroid occurs on the inner wall of the uterus between the muscle and endometrium. If this happens, you may be able to conceive but you'll continue to have miscarriages. Occasionally, a fibroid tumor may occur in such a location so as to block the fallopian tubes. If this happens, the tumors can be surgically removed.

Fibroid tumors are just one more complication that can occur with aging. However, just because you have fibroid tumors doesn't mean you'll have trouble conceiving. Even if you do find you are having problems conceiving, and you know you have fibroid tumors, surgery shouldn't be the first attempt at a solution. Both you and your partner should have a complete workup to try to identify any other possible source of infertility before resorting to a surgical treatment for fibroids.

Past Abortions

Many women worry that an abortion in the past may interfere with their ability to have a child in the future. By and large, this isn't true. Since abortions have been legalized, the procedure has become quite safe. If you had a legal abortion and experienced no complications afterward, then you are probably safe in assuming that you should have no difficulty conceiving as a result. If, however, you have had an illegal abortion, and especially if you developed an infection afterward, you would be at risk for having developed some scar tissue that could cause problems. If this is the case, be sure to tell your gynecologist about this history so that he will know what tests to perform to make sure your reproductive function is intact.

Male Problems

Now that you've scrutinized your medical history, you'll also want to scrutinize your partner's. If you don't have a man in your life at present, then simply take care to guard your own reproductive health. If you're currently married or otherwise involved, and know that you'll want to have children a few years down the road, then you should evaluate your partner's health for risks for infertility.

Past Illnesses

A primary illness that can affect a man's fertility is mumps, particularly if he contracted it during or after puberty. The mumps virus can attack the testicles and destroy the cells that produce sperm. If a man's testicles became sore when he was ill with the mumps, then this is a good clue that the virus reached those organs. If the infection was mild, the testicles may have recovered. But, if the infection was severe, there's a good chance that the sperm production cells were completely destroyed. Sometimes, though, just one testicle is attacked, which means that the man can still produce sperm.

Also, an infection in the epididymis—which, you may recall, houses the sperm until they mature—can cause scarring that keeps the sperm from exiting. The key symptom of this infection is a periodic painful swelling of the testicles.

Furthermore, if your partner has ever received chemotherapy or radiation therapy, particularly for cancer of the testicles, then there is a good chance that he has a decreased sperm count. After treatment for cancer, it can take four to five years for sperm counts to return to normal.

If your partner has had any one of these conditions, have him consult a urologist for an examination or a sperm analysis. A semen analysis is a simple, noninvasive, and relatively inexpensive test. Warn your partner in advance, though, that more than one semen analysis may be necessary.

Sperm counts can vary significantly from month to month under the most normal of circumstances. But, if your partner was exposed to something or had an illness that might have affected sperm production up to three months before the analysis, the results may be abnormal. The reason for this is that it takes about 74 days for a sperm to germinate and reach maturity, and another two weeks to pass through the testis and epididymis and appear in the ejaculate.[29] So, let's say your partner came down with a bad case of the flu and had a high fever in March. This high temperature could very well have damaged a significant number of his sperm. If so, it will be May before those damaged sperm begin to appear in his ejaculate. Although sperm production may return to normal after the fever disappears, it will be several more weeks before the healthy sperm appear in the ejaculate. For this same reason, even if your partner gives up activities that could be damaging his sperm—such as frequent, long soaks in the hot tub—it will take three to four months before his sperm count improves.

So, even if it takes a few trips to the doctor's office to obtain an accurate semen analysis, it will be worth it in the long run. If your partner is at risk for being infertile, it's better to discover that fact sooner rather than later.

Past Injuries

Carrying his reproductive organs outside his body makes a man especially prone to an injury in this area. Any sharp blow that caused him pain in his testicles, or caused his testicles to swell, could have caused some damage.

Another disorder that can cause dramatic and painful swelling is torsion. This is when the testicle spontaneously twists inside the scrotum. This cuts off the blood supply to the area and causes the testicle to react with pain and swelling. If the condition isn't corrected immediately, the testicle could die from lack of blood. To make matters worse, the dying testicle often causes antibodies to be sent to the other testicle, which can damage even the healthy testicle's ability to produce sperm. So, even if one testicle is left after such an event, it may not be able to produce viable sperm. Again, if this has occurred, have your partner consult a urologist for an evaluation. Or, if it occurs during your years of pregnancy postponement, he should seek emergency care from a urologist. Any delay could irreversibly damage the sperm production centers.

Past Surgery

Just as any surgical procedure on a woman's reproductive organs can impair her fertility, any surgery on or around a man's reproductive organs can affect his. This includes surgery to repair a hernia, which can bruise the ducts that carry sperm. Also, some men are born with a testicle that hasn't descended from the abdominal cavity into the scrotal sac. If this disorder isn't repaired at an early age, sterility can result. Even if it is repaired early on, it's possible for the ducts that carry the sperm to be damaged, resulting in a blockage from scar tissue.

If your partner needs to undergo any type of surgery that involves, or is near, his urinary tract or genital area during your years of postponement, you and your partner may want to talk with his doctor about the possibility of preserving some of your partner's sperm in a sperm bank before the procedure. This would be sort of an insurance policy. Just in case the surgery resulted in his no longer being able to produce sperm, you would have some of his sperm, frozen, which you could use during an artificial insemination procedure at a later date.

Medical Exam

And, as long as you're undergoing a medical exam to make sure that there aren't any unforeseen risks to your postponing pregnancy, your spouse or partner should do the same. After all, what good will it do for you to make sure that you're in prime shape to conceive if your spouse continues through the years with an undetected problem? This becomes even more important when you consider that the male is a major factor in a couple's infertility 40% of the time.

The first part of the exam will be to screen for illnesses that could affect his fertility. These include diabetes, thyroid problems, and renal disease. The doctor will also thoroughly check the genitals for any abnormality. One fairly common abnormality that can cause infertility is a varicocele.

A varicocele is a varicose vein in the testicle. Blood pools in this vein and increases the temperature in the testicle, thus killing sperm. Usually, the varicocele can be found during a physical examination. Sometimes more sophisticated measures are necessary to detect the abnormality, but these probably won't be used until it's certain there's a problem with sperm production. If a varicocele is found, it can be repaired by surgically tying off the vein. Not all varicoceles cause infertility, but as many as 30% of all men who are infertile have a varicocele. (Varicoceles are discussed in greater detail in Chapter 9.)

Another problem that the doctor may find is a hypospadias. This is when the opening at the end of the penis occurs on the underside of the penis rather than at the tip. This doesn't cause any problem until he and his partner try to become pregnant. A hypospadias contributes to infertility because the sperm are deposited too low in the vagina for enough of them to reach the cervix. To overcome this problem, the woman usually undergoes artificial insemination using her partner's sperm. This way, the sperm are manually deposited high in the uterus, thereby increasing the chances for conception to occur.

While your partner is with his doctor, he should ask him about any medications he is currently taking. Some medications can directly interfere with the production of sperm. Some of the more common culprits include antidepressant and antipsychotic medications as well as drugs taken for stomach problems, such as cimetidine, or for high blood pressure.

Conclusion

The goal of all of these steps is simply to protect your reproductive potential. While, at first glance, this may seem like a lot to be concerned with, it's really not. All we are really talking about are two things. The first is recognizing, and treating, any health problems you may have now that could affect your fertility in the future. The second is maintaining a healthful life-style through your years of postponement.

At times you may be tempted to discard all of this advice and simply live your life and take your chances. Quitting smoking, undergoing an annual gynecological exam, or even foregoing the convenience of an IUD may seem like too much bother. But I urge you to think again. With every year that you postpone, your risk for developing a problem that will lead to infertility increases. And the inconvenience of these steps is nothing compared to the inconvenience of an infertility examination, which we'll discuss in a later chapter.

6

Maximizing Your Chances for Conception

Once you decide to conceive, you'll no doubt want to accomplish your goal as quickly as possible. While this is true for almost any woman, it is especially true for women who have postponed childbearing. With age and possibly other risk factors plotting against you, you'll want to use every means available to maximize your chances for becoming pregnant. Following are some of the steps you can take to help you achieve your goal as quickly as possible.

Time Intercourse Appropriately

The first step in conceiving quickly is to make sure that you're having sex at the time in which you're most likely to conceive. Remember that the egg is only available for fertilization for 12 to 24 hours. If you miss that small window of opportunity, you'll have to delay your plans for pregnancy for at least one more month.

It's obvious, then, that you'll need to pinpoint, as closely as you can, the exact time of your ovulation. Most women assume that they ovulate in the middle of their menstrual cycle; but, this isn't necessarily true. Typically, ovulation occurs 14 days *before* the beginning of menstruation. Let's say your period starts on day 26 of your cycle. By counting backward 14 days, you can learn that you most likely ovulated on day 12. As you can see, only women who have 28-day cycles usually ovulate in the middle of the cycle, which would be day 14.

But, even if your cycle isn't a like-clockwork 28-day cycle, this doesn't mean there's a problem. Your cycle can range from 21 to 35 days and still be considered normal. At the same time, though, just because you have a regular menstrual period doesn't necessarily mean that you ovulate. You can menstruate month after month and still not ovulate. So, as you can see, simply "counting days" may not tell you much.

The only way to know for sure that you're ovulating is to have a series of ultrasound examinations performed. An ultrasound uses sound waves to create an image of an organ—in this case, your ovaries. Just before ovulation, the image will show several "blisters," or developing follicles, on your ovaries. These blisters continue to increase in size until at least one ruptures, presumably releasing an egg. The egg itself is too small to show up on ultrasound, but the image of a ruptured follicle is usually evidence enough that ovulation has occurred. Needless to say, ultrasound examinations aren't particularly practical. Luckily, there are more practical, and inexpensive, ways to discover when, or even if, you're ovulating.

One clue that you ovulate is if you experience certain premenstrual symptoms. These premenstrual symptoms may encompass a multitude of symptoms such as breast tenderness, water weight gain, irritability, headache, depression, and tension that begin about the time of ovulation and disappear around menstruation. Although you've probably always cursed this premenstrual time, these symptoms are actually a promising sign of ovulation. This is because premenstrual symptoms are linked to the same cyclic production of hormones that are needed for the production, and release, of an egg.

More definite ways of confirming ovulation include taking

your temperature, examining your cervical mucus, and using an ovulation predictor kit.

Basal Body Temperature

The simplest, and most inexpensive, way to gain some clue as to your ovulatory schedule is to take your temperature. The temperature of your body while you're at rest, called your basal body temperature, typically rises about a half a degree once ovulation has occurred and then remains elevated until the time of menstruation. This rise occurs because of the change in hormones that develops about the time of ovulation. As you may recall from Chapter 1, the hormone estrogen dominates the first half of the menstrual cycle, during which the endometrial lining develops and cervical mucus changes to become hospitable to sperm. Once ovulation occurs, the hormone progesterone enters the picture. It joins the hormone estrogen in seeing to it that the endometrial lining stays thick and rich in case a fertilized egg arrives. It's this increased production of progesterone that sends your temperature upward.

By taking your temperature, and plotting it on a graph, you'll be able to pinpoint when this temperature spike occurs. Then, in turn, you'll discover which days are your most fertile. And, besides helping you now, a temperature chart could help you in the future if you ever need to consult a fertility specialist. Most fertility doctors ask their patients to take their temperature, and record it on a chart, for several months as sort of a first step of an infertility workup. By maintaining such a chart from the beginning, not only will you be able to act on the evidence yourself, you'll be one step ahead in the evaluation process if you ever need to consult a doctor.

To keep an accurate chart, you must take your temperature every morning *before you get out of bed*. This means that you need to keep the thermometer and the chart on your nightstand where you can reach it without getting up. You should also try to take your temperature about the same time every day. It's really not important which kind of thermometer you use, although some are easier to use than others. A regular thermometer works just fine, but a basal thermometer is easier to read. Basal thermometers only record temperatures between 95 and 100 degrees and have marks for each tenth of a degree. You need to keep the thermometer in your mouth, and under your tongue, for about 5 minutes to obtain an accurate temperature. This can be difficult to accomplish, especially first thing in the morning when you're drowsy and you keep dozing off. For this reason, you may wish to foot the extra expense and buy an electronic digital thermometer. Available at most drugstores, these thermometers flash an accurate numerical temperature in only 30 seconds.

Once you have your temperature reading, you need to plot it on a graph. Some thermometers, such as basal thermometers, come with blank graphs. Your doctor's office can probably also furnish you with a graph that's ready to fill in. Or, if you wish, you can make one yourself out of a piece of graph paper. To do so, simply turn the paper lengthwise and, across the top of the paper, label each graph square with a day of your cycle, beginning with the number 1. Keep in mind that these are the days of your cycle, not the days of the month. Day 1 would be the first day of your menstrual period. Then, along the left-hand side of the paper, list the degree numbers, beginning with 97.0 degrees and continuing, at 0.2-degree increments, to 99.0 degrees. If you wish, you can label the days of the month along the bottom of the graph. For example, if your period begins on August 12, then August 12 and day 1 would both occupy the same square, with day 2 being August 13, and so on.

Then, every morning after you take your temperature, plot the temperature on the graph by placing a dot next to the corresponding temperature and underneath the appropriate day. Indicate the days on which you had sexual intercourse by drawing a circle around the dot for that day. Also make a note if something happened that would have altered your body temperature—for instance, if you were ill, or if you had a restless night.

Finally, indicate your days of menstruation by marking an "x" through the dots of the appropriate days.

After you've completed one cycle, examine your chart closely. If your temperature continued along at about the same level, except for a few minor variations, until approximately midcycle, at which time it suddenly rose by a half of a degree or more and then remained there, then this is a good indication that you ovulated. (See Figure 2.) But, if your temperature remained at about the same level for the entire month, with no identifiable and sustained increase, then this suggests that you may not have ovulated. (See Figure 3.) And finally, if your temperature rose, but then started to decline a few days before menstruation, then you may have a luteal phase defect. (This disorder will be covered in more detail in Chapter 8.) Another signal of a luteal phase defect is if your temperature didn't remain elevated for at least 10 to 12 days.

The major disadvantage of using the temperature chart to determine when to schedule intercourse is that the temperature doesn't rise until *after* ovulation has occurred. Occasionally, the temperature will dip to its lowest point just before the temperature spike; this dip is probably when ovulation occurs. Of course, it's difficult to know this at the time. Instead of trying to second-guess whether each slight dip in temperature is signaling ovulation, you should think of the charts as simply recording the *trends* of your cycle. For example, after you've taken your temperature for several months, can you say that the graphs all look similar, with the spike coming about the same time each month? If so, then you will probably be able to predict your approximate day of ovulation in future cycles. On the other hand, do your charts simply show minor variations in temperature, with no definite peak and sustained elevation? If this is the case, you may not be ovulating and you'd want to consult your doctor right away.

You need to know, though, that a temperature spike about midcycle and a sustained elevation does not prove, without a shadow of a doubt, that ovulation has occurred. Along that

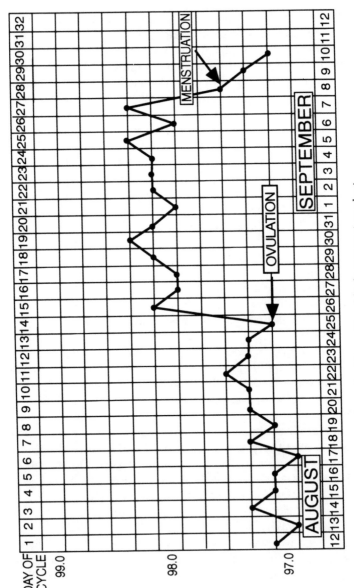

Figure 2.   Normal basal body temperature chart.

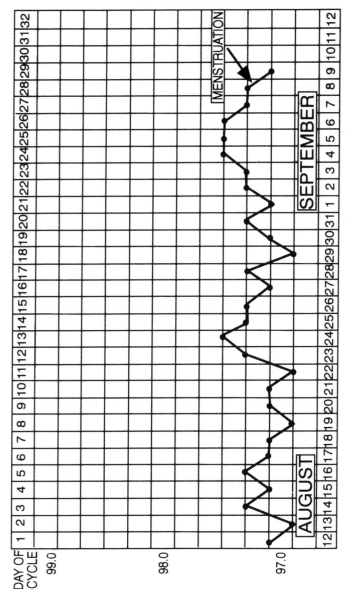

Figure 3.   Basal body temperature chart suggesting an absence of ovulation.

same line, a temperature chart that shows no temperature spike at all doesn't prove that ovulation hasn't occurred. As was stated earlier, an ultrasound is about the only way to know for certain that you're ovulating. But, a temperature chart can give very strong clues about when or even if you're ovulating. For most couples, this information can be extremely helpful. If you've taken and recorded your temperature faithfully for three to four months and you find that the temperature spike is consistent from month to month, you may wish to dispense with the temperature taking and simply schedule sex around this time period.

Cervical Mucus Examination

Another way to gain evidence about when you ovulate is to examine your cervical mucus. As you know, the cervix normally produces a thick and opaque mucus to discourage bacteria from entering the fragile environment of your reproductive tract. But besides discouraging bacteria, the mucus also thwarts the entry of sperm. So, just before ovulation, when the levels of estrogen and progesterone surge higher, the cervix ceases its normal production of mucus and begins to produce a thin, clear, and elastic mucus that sperm love. The only time this distinctive mucus is produced is around the time of ovulation. Therefore, if you can recognize this change in mucus, you will be able to identify your fertile period with more accuracy.

To examine the mucus, insert one or two fingers into your vagina and remove a small amount of mucus. Examine the color and consistency of the mucus, and then tap your forefinger against your thumb to determine how elastic it is. During your fertile time, the mucus is quite elastic and will stretch between your fingers. Repeat this process at several different times of the month so that you can distinguish between the different types of mucus. Once you see that the mucus has changed from being thick and opaque to being thin, clear, and elastic, you'll know that ovulation is about to occur.

Ovulation Predictor Kits

The newest, and perhaps the simplest, way to determine your time of ovulation is by using an ovulation predictor kit. Perhaps the best thing about these kits is that they identify this time *in advance*.

Available in most drugstores, these kits predict ovulation by detecting the presence of the hormone LH in urine. As you'll recall, LH surges some time in the middle of the menstrual cycle, causing the egg to burst from the ovary. The key to these kits is that LH surges *before* ovulation. The hormone rises first in the bloodstream and then spills over into the urine, making itself detectable about 20 to 40 hours before ovulation occurs. Therefore, once you can identify the hormone in your urine, you'll know that ovulation is pending.

These kits are relatively easy to use. They vary somewhat in technique, but, basically, they all require you to mix a sample of your urine with a couple of different chemicals. While timing each step, you apply the urine–chemical mixture to some device—such as a special pad or stick—which changes color when LH is present. Some kits, like OvuQuick and OvuGen, take only 3 to 4 minutes to perform. However, some doctors have found that some women may not be able to detect a surge using such quick kits, and instead recommend using kits such as OvuKit or OvuStick, which take 1 hour to perform.

Because the LH surge usually occurs in the morning between 5:00 and 9:00 AM, it's best to gather a urine specimen in the afternoon or early evening. Because LH appears in the bloodstream first, waiting until the afternoon gives the hormone time to spill over into your urine.[1] Alcohol, foods, and commonly used medications such as aspirin and Tylenol don't affect test results. However, danazol, birth control pills, and other types of hormones will affect the results.

Obviously, the best thing about ovulation predictor kits is that they can accurately let you know—in advance—when you will ovulate. A disadvantage, besides the inconvenience of kits that take an hour to complete, is the cost. On average, the kits cost from $30 to $60, depending upon the number of "tests" the kits contains. If your cycle is fairly regular, it's possible to make some kits last for two cycles. However, if your period is irregular, you may have to test your urine for several days to make sure that you catch your LH surge. If this is the case, you'll use more of the individual tests, and the cost will be higher.

Scheduling Sexual Intercourse

Now that you have an idea when you ovulate, when, exactly, is the best time to have sex? In general, the best way to arrange a meeting of egg and sperm is to have sex every 36 to 48 hours for 3 to 4 days before you expect to ovulate. Then, once you've ovulated, have sex at the same interval for the next 2 to 3 days. If you need to skip some of these days, it's better to skip the days following, rather than before, ovulation. The reason for this is that, almost as soon as you've ovulated, the rich, nourishing mucus in your cervix will begin to disappear. As a result, sperm aren't as likely to enter the uterus and climb up into the fallopian tubes. But, once the sperm are inside the hospitable confines of your cervix and fallopian tubes, they'll be able to hang around for a day or two. As a result, if you have sex before you ovulate, the sperm will be waiting when the egg pops out of the ovary and begins its cruise down the fallopian tube.

If you're using an ovulation predictor kit to predict your ovulation, it's probably a good idea to have sex as soon as you detect a surge. Keep in mind that, if you're only checking your urine once a day, it will have been 24 hours since you last checked. Therefore, it's possible that your surge started sometime during that intervening 24 hours. And, since ovulation occurs, on average, 35 hours after the onset of the surge, you may not have much time to lose.

It's also a good idea for men to refrain from ejaculating for a couple of days before your most fertile time. This will allow the sperm count to build up, giving you the best chance possible for conception. At the same time, though, don't overdo the abstinence bit. Abstaining for 7 days or more could actually hurt your chances. The reason for this is that sperm age like anything else and, after about 7 days, they may no longer be "top quality." And you wouldn't want these older sperm—which are less able to fertilize an egg—crowding out any of their younger and more viable counterparts.

You also probably shouldn't have sex any more often than every 36 to 48 hours during your fertile time. Ejaculation empties the epididymis of all available sperm, and it takes about 40 hours for the epididymis to refill with new sperm. Having sex more frequently than every 36 hours will just depress a man's sperm count. This may not be too harmful if your partner has a great sperm count but, if his count is at all marginal, having sex too frequently could hurt your chances for conception. Of course, spacing intercourse any further apart than every 48 hours could cause you to miss your fertile period entirely.

Wow, you might be saying, whatever happened to sex being fun and spontaneous? Sex can still be fun; in fact, you should make an effort to keep it so. But, unfortunately, when you're trying to conceive in the shortest amount of time possible, spontaneity gets sacrificed. At the same time, though, you don't have to conduct your sex life like a military exercise: day 11, sex in the evening; day 12, no sex; day 13, sex in the morning. Eventually, this is what it may boil down to as you try to maximize your chances for conception. But for now—at least at the beginning—try not to be so hard on yourself or your partner. Sex on command not only takes all the fun out of sex, it can actually foster sexual dysfunction. Remember that sperm can survive in your reproductive tract for a couple, or even several, days. Having sex every couple of days around the time of ovulation means that there will always be some sperm available when the egg finally begins its trip down the fallopian tube.

So try not to force the issue. You need to have sex during the right time period if you're ever going to get pregnant, of course; but, in the interim, try to keep your sex life as fun and stress-free as possible.

Use the Best Sexual Position

The next step in encouraging conception is to make sure that, during sexual intercourse, the sperm end up as high in your vagina and as close to your cervix as possible. The best position to facilitate this to have sex in a face-to-face position with the man on top. This position allows the sperm to pool high in the vagina and hastens their trip into the warm and nourishing environment of the cervix.

To further enhance your chances, tell your partner not to withdraw abruptly. In addition, you should remain lying down for 30 minutes after sex. You may also want to elevate your buttocks on a couple of pillows for that time. The most important thing, though, is not to pop right up out of bed. You want to help the sperm along as much as possible, and, if you stand up right after sex, you risk losing some of the ejaculate through drainage. After 30 minutes, though, feel free to get up if you want to. Any sperm that haven't made it to the cervix by that time will never make it.

Avoid Douching and Lubricants

Again, your purpose here is to do everything possible to encourage the sperm on their journey up through your reproductive system. Of course, if you douche immediately after having sex, then you would be washing away much-needed sperm. Besides that, douching after your menstrual period or at any other time in your cycle can create more problems with your reproductive system than it cures.

To begin with, douching is *not* necessary for cleanliness and good hygiene. The vagina lubricates and cleanses itself; in fact, douching washes away these beneficial lubricants. Even worse, women who douche regularly have twice the risk of having an ectopic pregnancy as compared to women who don't douche at all.[2] Doctors believe this occurs because the act of douching washes bacteria from the vagina up into the uterus and fallopian tubes. And, as you already know, an infection in the fallopian tubes can lead to scar tissue and blockages, which, in turn, can lead to an ectopic pregnancy.

The only time you should douche is if your doctor recommends a specific douche preparation to treat a certain medical condition. Otherwise, the best course is to allow your reproductive system to cleanse itself.

Besides not douching, you should also avoid using lubricants during sexual intercourse. Even common lubricants, such as K-Y jelly or petroleum jelly, may either kill sperm or, at the very least, interfere with their movement. Really, this is only common sense. Imagine what it would be like if *you* had to swim through petroleum jelly. If you must use a lubricant, use egg white or vegetable oil, which aren't toxic to sperm. However, don't use saliva, which can interfere with fertilization.

Avoid High Temperatures

For sperm to be produced, they need an environment that is about four degrees cooler than the temperature in the rest of the body. Therefore, anything that substantially raises the temperature of a man's genitals can interfere with fertility. The first situation that can cause this to occur is if the testicles have never descended into the scrotal sac. This condition occurs in about one out of every 200 births. Optimally, it should be repaired before the child is 2 or 3 years old. If it's not repaired, infertility can result because the temperature of the abdominal cavity is too high for sperm to be produced.

Even if the testicles have descended into the scrotal sac, it's still possible to raise the temperature of the testicles to a level that would impair sperm production. One way to do this is by lounging in a hot tub, sauna, or hot bath. The water in most hot tubs remains between 101 and 103 degrees; as you can see, this is well above the 94 or 95 degrees that sperm need to thrive.

Therefore, if your partner soaks in a hot tub on a regular basis, your chances of conception could be impaired.

Likewise, wearing tight underwear or pants that bind the testicles close to the body can also raise testicular temperature and lower sperm counts. The same thing goes for wearing a jock strap or athletic supporter too often. The most obvious solution to this problem is for your partner to avoid these activities while you're trying to get pregnant. He should make his hot showers or baths brief, and avoid soaking in a hot tub or steaming in a sauna. In addition, it's also a good idea, especially if he has a marginal sperm count, to forsake tight underwear for boxer shorts.

Another possible source of damaging high temperatures that many couples overlook is the man's work environment. One profession that exposes its workers to excessive temperatures for prolonged periods is truck driving. Truck drivers sit for hours at a time on the hot seat of a truck cab; the hot temperature of the seat can raise the temperature in the testicles to a level that could impair sperm production. Also, welders who work inside tight spaces, such as storage tanks, may be exposed to temperatures up to 120 degrees. Again, this is too high for optimum sperm production.

High temperatures are more of a concern for men while you're trying to conceive. But, once conception occurs, you also need to watch the thermometer. Exposing yourself to the same high temperatures after you've conceived can damage a developing embryo. This means that you should also avoid things like hot tubs. At least one large study has shown that soaking in a hot tub during the first six weeks of pregnancy could increase your risk for having a baby with spina bifida or a brain defect by as much as two to three times.

Remember, after your fertile time, there will be at least a two-week lag during which you won't know whether or not you're pregnant. The best course of action is to treat that time as if you were pregnant so that you don't do anything to jeopardize your pregnancy.

Eliminate Interfering Medications

Certain medications—including antihypertensives, anti-depressants, corticosteroids (taken to decrease inflammation), and hallucinatory drugs—can impair the man's ability to produce sperm. Likewise, so can narcotics and marijuana. Even large doses of aspirin, if taken regularly, can inhibit sperm production.

If your partner must take certain medications because of a medical condition—for example, he has high blood pressure that must be controlled with medications—then ask him to talk with his doctor about the possibility of his particular medication causing a problem with infertility. If the drug can cause problems in that area, have your partner ask the doctor if he can be changed to another drug or treatment, at least temporarily.

Keep Exercise Moderate

The importance of exercising to keep your body in shape for a postponed pregnancy was discussed in the previous chapter. We also mentioned briefly that it's important not to overdo it. Now, don't take this as an excuse not to exercise at all. Regular exercise is important for your overall health and well-being. Just keep your exercise routine at a moderate level. Pushing it and exercising to excess could depress your level of fertility.

One disadvantage of intensive exercise is that it can elevate your body temperature to dangerously high levels. And, if you're in the early stages of pregnancy, the high temperature could harm the developing embryo, resulting in birth defects. But even before that would happen, regular intensive exercise could impair your ability to get pregnant.

A study by Harvard University of more than 5000 women found that intense physical activity interfered with the production of estrogen.[3] As you already know, your body needs a certain level of estrogen to be able to ovulate. These changes could happen despite that fact that you may continue to menstruate regularly. This means that you would have no outward sign that your reproductive system was being upset by your exercise routine; you just wouldn't be able to get pregnant. Luckily, infertility caused by exercise is reversible; once the intense workouts are discontinued, hormone secretion returns to normal.

If you have trouble conceiving, and you regularly participate in a fairly intensive exercise routine, then back off a little bit and see what happens. But don't take this as an excuse not to exercise for the entire time you are trying to conceive. All in all, the benefits of moderate workouts—including a lower risk of heart disease and cancer—far outweigh the dangers. And besides that, regular exercise can help you control one more factor that can influence fertility: stress.

Control Stress

There's no question that problems with infertility cause stress. But what no one knows for sure is whether stress causes, or contributes to, infertility. Even if you haven't had any evidence of being infertile, trying to conceive under a time clock can cause you to feel terrific stress. Most doctors will tell you that if you're not stressed out to the extent that you drop 20 pounds or stop menstruating, then your fertility will not be affected. But, this may not be completely true. Some experts are beginning to explore the theory that stress may, in fact, cause infertility.

When you are feeling stressed, your body thinks that it is under attack by very real, very tangible dangers. As a result, it kicks off what is known as the "fight or flight" response to try to protect itself. Besides causing your heart rate to speed up, your pupils to dilate, and your palms to sweat, it also alters the secretion of several of the hundreds of hormones and chemicals that keep your body running. In turn, altering the production level of some of these hormones, however slightly, may affect your reproductive function. For example, stress can cause you to have a deficiency of progesterone, which is vital to the reproductive process, or to have an elevated level of the hormone prolactin, which can disrupt ovulation.

Researchers know that stress can inhibit ovulation or cause your fallopian tubes to spasm, which could interfere with the safe transport of an egg. Stress can also interfere with the normal transport and implantation of a fertilized egg. But women aren't the only ones affected by stress. Men who are feeling the effects of stress may have a depressed sperm count, or they may suffer from sexual dysfunction.

With this in mind, some researchers have sought to improve fertility by helping people control their levels of stress. One such study, performed in conjunction with the New England Deaconess Hospital and Harvard Medical School, centered around 54 women who had been trying unsuccessfully to become pregnant for 3 years. These women and their husbands then participated in a 10-week program designed to help them alleviate stress. The program taught the couples how to elicit what is known as the relaxation response. Developed by Dr. Herbert Benson, the relaxation response is the process of mentally relaxing by using deep breathing, meditation, and positive mental imagery. What Dr. Benson found is that, once people completely relax through the use of these techniques, some very real physical changes result. These changes include a decreased heart rate, lowered blood pressure, slowed respiratory rate, and relaxed muscle tone. For this study, the couples completed questionnaires designed to measure their levels of stress both before and after the course. After completion of the course, every participant felt less depressed and less tense. But even more important, 18 (or 34%) of the participants became pregnant within 6 months of completing the program.[4] Keep in mind that these women had been trying, without success, for an average of 3 years to become pregnant.

Another study examined the anxiety levels of 42 women

with unexplained infertility. Twice a week for a year, each woman received an evaluation designed to measure her level of
situational anxiety—which is simply the anxiety a person feels
as a result of life circumstances. During the year when the women were being evaluated, 12 of the 42 women became pregnant. What's interesting is that the researchers found that the
women who became pregnant were more likely to have had a
decrease in the amount of stress they were experiencing in their
everyday lives. Furthermore, they found that the women who
were suffering from greater levels of situational anxiety were
much less likely to become pregnant. Every woman who became pregnant showed a decrease in situational anxiety before
pregnancy.

But the study didn't end there. It further selected 14 women
who still hadn't become pregnant and then randomly divided
those into two groups of seven. One group received no treatment. The second group underwent a 16-session individual behavioral treatment program that taught them, among other
things, how to elicit the relaxation response and how to restruc-
ture their thinking patterns. By the end of the 3-month project,
four of the seven experimental patients had become pregnant.
None of the control patients conceived.[5]

The results from both of these studies are preliminary; there
was no control group, so we can't bank on the results. There is
nothing *definite* about whether, or how, stress affects fertility. But
the results certainly do seem to indicate that the amount of
stress you're experiencing in everyday life can affect your level
of fertility. Therefore, try not to put yourself too much under the
gun. Maximize your chances for conception by following the
guidelines in this chapter. Then, at least for awhile, let nature
take its course. Remember, conception can take time. Of course,
if you have any sign of a physical problem, consult your gynecologist right away.

Whether you end up seeing a doctor or not, you would no
doubt benefit from relaxation training. Investigate sources in
your community—such as colleges, community centers, or hos-

pital well-patient centers—for courses on meditation or on other relaxation techniques. Learning to relax and slow down the internal pace of your body's functions will not only improve your overall health—it just may help you conceive.

Shape Up Your Lifestyle

If you didn't make it a point to quit smoking during your years of postponement, then you need to do so immediately. Now that you're trying to conceive, giving up cigarettes is more important than ever. If the hazards of smoking discussed in the previous chapter didn't sway you, then the point is worth reemphasizing. Smoking decreases your chances for becoming pregnant. It also increases your risk for having an ectopic pregnancy and can alter the normal development of the embryo. Consider this: nicotine is ten times more concentrated in uterine fluid than it is in the bloodstream.[6] That means that you are literally bathing your newly developing embryo in nicotine. And if that's not enough, smoking reduces sperm density, which could cause you to take longer to conceive.

Along with quitting smoking, now is the time when you need to keep close tabs on your alcohol intake. This is especially true during those two weeks every month when you don't know if you're pregnant or not. The same reasons not to drink that were discussed in the previous chapter apply here. Drinking heavily while pregnant can have disastrous results, that's a given. But drinking only moderately can also affect the fetus. So why take the chance? If you've waited this long to have a baby, why even risk the possibility of trading a few of your infant's IQ points for a couple of glasses of wine? While the wine may not measurably damage the embryo, it certainly won't help it.

Finally, this is also the time to make sure that you're eating a balanced diet. You need to be consuming an adequate amount of carbohydrates, proteins, and fats along with a sufficient amount of vitamins and minerals. Talk with your doctor about the possibility of taking prenatal vitamins now, before you conceive. Remember what we talked about in the previous chapter: your nutritional status before you conceive can influence the development of the embryo.

Additional Points to Consider

Finally, if you don't become pregnant as quickly as you thought you would, the time of year may have something to do with it. It's a known fact that fewer babies are born in the spring, which means that fewer people conceive during the summer months.

Intrigued by these statistics, epidemiologist Richard J. Levine led a study to determine why this was true. The study, which was conducted at the Chemical Industry Institute of Toxicology at Research Triangle Park in North Carolina, examined semen samples of 131 men who worked outdoors in San Antonio, Texas. What they found was that, during the summer, all of the men experienced a decreased sperm count. In fact, both the density and the number of sperm in the semen samples were 25 to 30% lower than were the samples from the same men during the winter.[7]

Ah, you say, of course sperm counts go down in the summer; that's because it's so hot. But that doesn't seem to be the sole reason. If it were, researchers would have found that the men who had the most depressed sperm counts worked the greatest number of hours outdoors. But that wasn't the case. Furthermore, studies in France and Switzerland have produced the same results, and summers in those countries aren't nearly as hot as the summers in San Antonio. You need to know, though, that other studies have not shown this change. Even so, the possibility is worth considering.

Now, this doesn't mean that you won't be able to conceive during the summer. If that were true, no one would have a birthday in May. Just keep in mind that if you're trying to conceive in the summer, there's a chance that it will take longer. Also keep this in mind if your husband undergoes a sperm count during the summer. If his count is slightly low, rather than panic, just have the count repeated during the fall or winter.

Conclusion

In conclusion, there's nothing wrong with trying to nudge mother nature along in your quest for pregnancy. After determining your time of ovulation, schedule intercourse at appropriate intervals both before and after that time. Encourage the meeting of an egg and sperm by remaining in bed for a time after sex and by not douching or using lubricants. Also, help your spouse keep his sperm count high by identifying any interfering medications and by having him avoid high temperatures. But most of all, try to keep your sex life as fun and as spontaneous as possible. If you feel your anxiety level rising, perform stress-reduction exercises and continue to include exercise as a part of your daily routine. Above anything else, this should be an exciting and memorable part of your life; this is the time when you and your partner have decided to expand your family.

7

Consulting an Expert

After you've been trying, perhaps unsuccessfully, to become pregnant for several months, you may begin to wonder if you should consult an expert. On the one hand, you know that it can simply take time to become pregnant, especially if you're older. What's more, you don't want to endure the emotional trauma, or incur the expense, of an infertility workup if it's not necessary. But, on the other hand, you don't want to waste valuable time if something is wrong. So, how do you know when you've tried long enough, and it's time to get professional help?

Deciding When to Seek Help

Unfortunately, there's no definite answer as to when you should seek expert advice. Infertility doesn't have any symptoms, like pain or a fever, to alert you to its presence. As a result, some women try for years to become pregnant, never knowing that their fallopian tubes are completely blocked. At the same time, other women endure the intense process of an infertility workup only to learn that there is nothing wrong.

The best time to consult a doctor varies with each woman. As a general rule of thumb, though, if you're over age 35 and have been timing intercourse appropriately for six months without getting pregnant, then it would be a good idea for you to go ahead and visit your doctor for an evaluation. There's no need to panic at this point, though. Remember, as was discussed in Chapter 2, a significant percentage of normally fertile women over age 35 won't become pregnant after even a year of trying. But, by seeking help sooner rather than later, you won't be wasting any time if something is wrong that can be remedied.

However, if you know, or at least suspect, that you have a problem with fertility, then, by all means, consult an expert as soon as possible. For example, if you think that you may have endometriosis, if you have a history of pelvic infections, if you used an IUD, or if your mother took DES while she was pregnant with you, then you may wish to receive an evaluation sooner rather than later. The same thing goes if your partner has had a scrotal injury or had mumps after the onset of puberty. Review Chapter 5, "Maintaining Your Fertility"; if you violated several of those "golden rules" for prolonged fertility, you may wish to see a doctor early in the process of your quest for pregnancy. Also, take the preconception questionnaire located in Appendix A; the information found there may also help you know if you're at risk for being infertile.

What Could Be Wrong?

In most instances, a couple's infertility isn't related to one particular abnormality. Rather, it's caused by a number of different factors. Taken separately, none of these factors would be significant enough to cause a problem. But, when added together, they can disrupt the reproductive process and prevent pregnancy.

Of course, these disruptive factors can occur in a man's reproductive system, or in a woman's. A man's reproductive responsibilities are fairly straightforward. Basically, he's charged with manufacturing sperm and then delivering an adequate number of motile sperm into a woman's vagina at the appropriate time. In contrast, the task of a woman's reproductive system is much more varied. Not only must it produce eggs, it must deliver those eggs to the uterus, which, in turn, must be up to the task of holding and nourishing the embryo as it develops into a baby. An abnormality in just one of these areas could be enough to cause infertility.

That's where knowing, in general, about the types of things that could be wrong can help you decide when, or even if, you need to consult a doctor. Furthermore, thoroughly searching your health and history for any hint of a problem before you ever consult a doctor will allow you to go to that first visit armed with specific, pertinent information about your reproductive health. This information could be the key that allows the doctor to hone in on any problem areas quickly and easily.

Of course, many factors causing infertility require a medical evaluation to detect. But there are many other infertility problems that send out signals that you may be able to discern. Keep in mind that the purpose of this chapter isn't to discuss everything that could be wrong with your reproductive system. Rather, it's to point out some of the most common problems and to highlight some of the clues that may alert you to the existence of a problem. Some clues will sound familiar. For example, in the previous chapter, you learned to watch your body's signals to pinpoint your time of ovulation. But now it's time to get more specific in your search. Although it's never a pleasant task to consider that something might be wrong, the sooner you identify a problem, the sooner you'll be on your way toward resolving it.

Ovarian Factors

As you already know, the ovaries are responsible for producing eggs. Not ovulating at all, or at least not ovulating regularly, is a problem for about 25% of the couples undergoing an infertility evaluation. It's obvious that if you don't ovulate, you can't become pregnant. But it's also important to ovulate regularly, especially when you consider that—even under the most ideal circumstances—you have only about a 30% chance for becoming pregnant within any given month. So, if you're only ovulating three or four times a year, it could take years to get pregnant.

Many, many factors can disrupt ovulation. The most common factors are excessive weight loss or gain (although a loss or gain of as little as five pounds can temporarily disrupt ovulation), excessive exercise, and extreme emotional stress. The good news, though, is that you can control these influences. Simply maintain your ideal body weight (although in cases of severe obesity or anorexia, you may need to seek professional help to do so), limit your exercise routine, and take steps to reduce your stress level, such as enrolling in a stress reduction class.

But other factors—factors over which you may not have any control—can also affect ovulation. One cause is a disorder called polycystic ovarian syndrome, a complex disorder where the ovarian follicles don't regularly release eggs. Other causes of ovulatory disorders include chronic illness, hormonal imbalances (including too little progesterone or an excess of male hormone), an over- or underactive thyroid gland, seizure disorders, or even approaching menopause. To assess and treat these factors, you'd have to seek medical help. But, the first step is recognizing there's a problem. Many times, a woman's body sends out signals as to whether or not she's ovulating properly. Knowing what to look for could help you identify an ovulatory problem early in your attempts at becoming pregnant.

To determine whether you're ovulating regularly, think about your menstrual cycle. Do you menstruate regularly? Do you experience premenstrual symptoms? If you do, then you're most likely ovulating, although, of course, this is no guarantee. In addition, if your back and legs ache and your breasts become sore just before your period starts, then this, too, is a reassuring sign; these muscle cramps are caused by the same peaking and withdrawal of progesterone that accompany ovulation. An even greater assurance of ovulation is if you feel a slight pain in your left or right abdominal side about the time ovulation should be occurring. This pain, called *mittelschmerz*, occurs when the egg breaks free from the ovarian follicle. If you don't feel this pain, though, don't worry. Many normal, ovulating women don't feel it either.

The next step in determining whether or not you're ovulating as you should is to analyze your basal body temperature chart. As was discussed earlier, your temperature should rise about a half of a degree somewhere in the middle of your cycle (or 14 days before your next period starts) and then remain elevated until you begin menstruation. If it does, then this is further reassuring evidence that you are indeed ovulating.

A sign that you may not be ovulating, though, is if you don't feel any symptoms either before or during your period. Most of the symptoms that accompany a menstrual cycle occur because of the peaking and withdrawal of estrogen and progesterone. If these hormones remain in a steady state instead of cycling like they're supposed to, you won't feel any symptoms, *and* you won't be producing eggs. Other signs of ovulatory trouble include changes in the length or regularity of your menstrual cycle, changes in the amount of your menstrual flow, and even changes in your appearance.

Cycle Regularity

A normal menstrual cycle ranges between 24 and 32 days. Cycles that are significantly shorter or longer than this norm could indicate that something's amiss. This is especially true if your periods are erratic; for example, one month you may menstruate after 35 days, but then, the next month, your period may start after only 21 days. Because it's the act of ovulation that sets the date for the beginning of menstruation, erratic cycles often signal that ovulation isn't occurring.

To explain further, you may recall that the hormones your reproductive system needs to operate are produced by the hypothalamus and pituitary, which reside in the brain, as well as by the ovaries. When ovulation occurs, the corpus luteum—which is the site from which the egg ovulated—secretes the hormones estradiol and progesterone during the last half of the menstrual cycle. If the egg isn't fertilized, the corpus luteum shrinks, the hormone levels plummet, and menstruation occurs. But, if ovulation doesn't occur, the corpus luteum never makes an appearance. Without the corpus luteum, progesterone does not surge and decline, and the endometrium is never quite sure when to slough off. As a result, the endometrium breaks down at different times instead of all at once and menstruation becomes irregular. Other factors that can stop ovulation include anything that interferes with the production of hormones by the centers in the brain, or that alters how the ovaries respond to these hormones. Such factors include recent birth control pill use, tumors of the pituitary gland, or even the use of certain drugs, such as tranquilizers.

Women at both ends of the spectrum of menstruation—including young women just beginning to menstruate and women approaching menopause—tend to have irregular periods, which means they're probably not ovulating regularly. Not all women approaching menopause have irregular periods, though. Some continue to have regular cycles, but the length of the cycle just gets shorter and shorter. For example, instead of menstruating every 28 days, they begin to menstruate every 26, or even every 25 days. The reason for this abbreviated cycle is that the first half of the cycle, called the follicular phase, which is responsible for causing the egg to mature, grows shorter. As a result, even if ovulation does occur, the egg may not have had enough time in which to mature and, therefore, isn't a likely candidate for fertilization.

Type of Flow

Besides being regular, the flow from your period should also be consistent. For example, your period should last about three to five days, with the flow being heavier during the first couple of days and then tapering off to spotting by the last day. If this describes your period, then your body is most likely producing hormones as it should. But, if your flow is excessively heavy, or if it tends to be light for several months and then becomes quite heavy for a month, then you may have a hormone imbalance or a uterine abnormality.

As you already know, the hormone progesterone makes its appearance in the latter half of the menstrual cycle. Among its other responsibilities, progesterone softens the endometrial lining that accumulated during the first half of the cycle. Not only does this make the endometrium a welcoming surface in which a fertilized egg can bed down, it also gives the endometrium a texture that is likely to slough off cleanly and completely if fertilization doesn't occur. It's important that the old endometrium shed completely at the end of each cycle so that the uterus can regenerate a smoothly uniform endometrium the next month.

If your body doesn't produce enough progesterone, the endometrium won't soften appropriately. And if it doesn't soften appropriately, it won't shed evenly when the time comes. Instead, it will break off in chunks, leaving remnants behind. Then, when the endometrium begins to build the next month, it will build on top of these remnants, causing an excessive and uneven buildup. This typically results in a flow that is heavy, or one that is light for a couple of months and then excessive for a month. You might experience some spotting in between periods as the endometrium struggles to rid itself of excess tissue. (You also need to be aware that spotting between periods can signal problems other than those relating to ovulation. For example, spotting could also be a sign of a cervical or uterine disorder. For this reason, if you consistently spot between periods, you should consult your doctor for an evaluation.)

Considering all of this, and knowing that progesterone is a key player in the ovulatory process, it's possible that, if you're short on progesterone, you're not ovulating appropriately. Even if you are continuing to ovulate, but you're not producing enough progesterone, your uterus won't be a habitable environment for a fertilized egg.

Progesterone isn't the only hormone that can disrupt the delicate timing of ovulation and otherwise alter your menstrual flow. Thyroid hormone can do the same. The thyroid gland, which resides in the hollow of your neck, secretes thyroid hormone. The chief responsibility of thyroid hormone is to control your body's metabolic rate. If this gland is overactive, and produces too much hormone, or if it is underactive, and doesn't produce enough, the hormonal equilibrium achieved between your hypothalamus, pituitary gland, and ovaries can be completely thrown off balance. In turn, this could disrupt ovulation and alter the quality of your menstrual flow.

Other signs of an overly active thyroid gland include excessive hunger, eating large amounts of food without gaining weight, nervousness, irritability, and feeling hot and sweaty. Conversely, a gland that isn't producing enough thyroid hormone causes weight gain (even with low caloric intake), fatigue, and sensitivity to cold. A chief clue as to whether or not you should be on the lookout for such a problem to develop is if someone in your family has thyroid disease. This disorder tends to run in families, so if either of your parents, any of your aunts and uncles, or your siblings have a thyroid problem, then you, too, could be at risk. If you have any of these symptoms, check with your doctor. A simple blood test is usually enough to determine whether your thyroid gland is functioning normally.

Still another hormone that can throw a wrench into the ovulatory works is prolactin. Prolactin, which is normally produced by the pituitary gland during and following pregnancy, stimulates the production of breast milk. It also happens to disrupt ovulation. Occasionally, a woman's body may produce prolactin even though she's not pregnant. When that happens, ovulation stops. Sometimes, an elevated prolactin level may not produce any symptoms; at other times, though, it causes the woman's nipples to secrete a milky discharge.

Appearance

Another sign as to whether or not you're ovulating normally could be contained in your appearance. For example, some women who don't ovulate secrete an increased amount of a male hormone that can cause subtle changes in appearance. This doesn't mean they're any less of a woman. All women secrete a certain amount of male hormones. It's just that, occasionally, the production of the hormone can get out of hand.

Physical signs that an excess amount of male hormone is being produced include an increased growth of facial hair, especially on the jaw, chin, or upper lip; a small amount of hair on the breast; increased pubic hair that rises into the midline of the abdomen; and hair on the great toe. Another common sign of excess male hormone production is oily skin and acne, especially acne that persists beyond the teenage years. Only in extreme cases will severe masculine changes occur.

*   *   *

If you have any of these signs of impaired ovulation—either a temperature chart without a temperature spike, irregular periods, abnormal flow, or abnormal hair growth and acne—then you should consult a doctor right away. Of course, even if you don't have any of these trouble signs, there's no guarantee that you're ovulating normally. But, then again, the chances are good that you are.

Fallopian Tube Factors

The next organs that you need to consider when evaluating the effectiveness of your reproductive system are your fallopian tubes. Going hand-in-hand with your fallopian tubes is the state of your peritoneum. The peritoneum is the tissue that lines the inside of your abdominal cavity and surrounds your reproductive organs. Anything that disrupts this delicate environment—such as trauma, surgery, or infection—can cause the peritoneum to scar. In turn, this scar tissue can create all kinds of havoc with the functioning of your reproductive system, especially with your fallopian tubes.

The key to understanding how peritoneal factors—which are uncovered in about 25% of the women who undergo infertility evaluations—can affect your chances for pregnancy, you need to appreciate the complexity of the fallopian tube's function. The fallopian tube is more than a tube down which the egg travels on its way to the uterus. The fallopian tubes are, in fact, complex structures. First of all, the fallopian tube must reach up to catch the egg as it pops from the ovary. Then, once it has the egg safely in its grasp, the fallopian tube actively works to propel the egg onward toward the uterus. What's particularly remarkable is that the fallopian tube is able to propel the egg *down* the tube at the same time it's encouraging the sperm to move *up* the tube. Next, besides providing the spot for fertilization, the fallopian tube safely houses and nourishes the developing embryo until it can alight in the waiting uterus.

Based on these sketchy facts about the fallopian tube's functions, it's easy to see that clear, functioning fallopian tubes are essential for conception. Scar tissue inside the peritoneum can wrap around the fallopian tubes, constricting them so that an egg can't pass. At the very least, scar tissue can bind the tubes, preventing them from reaching up to catch an egg as it bursts from the ovary. If that happens, the egg will simply plummet to the depths of the abdominal cavity, carrying with it all hopes for fertilization.

You're at risk for having scar tissue put a kink in your plans for motherhood if you've ever had abdominal or pelvic surgery, an abdominal injury, a ruptured appendix, or pelvic inflammatory disease. As was discussed in Chapter 5, PID as a result of *Chlamydia* infection can be particularly devastating, causing irreversible damage to the reproductive organs of women who may have no idea they've had an infection.[1] Additional causes of peritoneal scarring include endometriosis, which was also discussed in detail in Chapter 5, or IUD use. In fact, if you've used an

IUD, your chances for having peritoneal scarring are four times greater than those of a woman who never used the device.[2]

Also, besides the danger of scar tissue, it's possible for fallopian tubes to be deformed. Women whose mothers took DES while pregnant are particularly prone to having malformed—and malfunctioning—fallopian tubes. In fact, women who have deformed fallopian tubes as a result of DES exposure have a risk that's five times greater than normal for having an ectopic pregnancy.[3]

Often, the only real symptom of peritoneal scarring is infertility. As a result, short of a medical evaluation, you may not be able to determine whether or not you're afflicted. Your best clue may come through closely evaluating your medical history. Have you ever had PID? Have you used an IUD? Have you had several sexual partners? Have you ever had an abdominal injury, abdominal surgery, or a ruptured appendix? If so, then you should consult your doctor for a workup, mentioning specifically that you're concerned about your chances for having peritoneal scar tissue.

Cervical Factors

The next structure that needs to be functioning appropriately if you're to become pregnant is the cervix. Besides being the portal for the sperm's entry into the uterus and fallopian tubes, the mucus produced by the cervix protects and houses the sperm until they can depart on their journey toward fertilization. In addition, the cervical mucus weeds out weak or deformed sperm so that they don't interfere with the progress of their more viable companions. So, as you can see, an abnormality here, either in the structure of the cervix or in the quality or quantity of cervical mucus, could be a major stumbling block in your efforts to conceive. Even so, cervical factors are a cause of infertility less than 5% of the time.

One risk factor for a malfunctioning cervix is past cervical surgery. This can include cryosurgery and cone biopsies, a procedure in which a wedge of cervical tissue is removed. These surgical procedures can cause the cervix to scar and constrict, thus restricting the number of sperm that can enter the uterus, and can even destroy some of the glands that produce mucus.

Cervical scarring, and a resultant constricted opening, can also result from abortions and D & Cs (dilatation and curettage). Besides this, these same procedures can weaken the cervix, causing it to become flaccid. A weak or flaccid cervix won't be able to support the weight of a developing fetus. When the weight increases beyond a certain point, the cervix will give way, resulting in a miscarriage or premature delivery.

Other possible cervical abnormalities include some that are easy to remedy—such as cervical infections—and some that aren't—such as deformities. Cervical infections can interfere with pregnancy because the infectious process produces white blood cells, which can actually attack and kill sperm. If an infection is allowed to continue unchecked, it can even destroy some of the glands that produce mucus. Fortunately, antibiotics can usually clear up the infection. So, if you have any symptoms of an infection—such as a chronic vaginal discharge or spotting—call your gynecologist for treatment.

Cervical deformities, on the other hand, aren't quite so easy to cure. You're particularly at risk for having an abnormally shaped cervix if your mother took DES while she was pregnant with you. This deformity may not interfere with your chances for pregnancy, but it could increase your risk for having a miscarriage.[4]

And finally, you might be contributing to, or even causing, a cervical problem if you douche or use vaginal lubricants during intercourse. Douching not only washes away sperm, it also washes away the all-important cervical mucus. Lubricants cause problems because they can interfere with the movement of sperm. The problems caused by douching or lubricants are the easiest ones to solve: simply stop both practices, and your cervix should return to normal.

Your doctor should be able to identify some cervical problems—including infections and some deformities—through a simple vaginal examination. Other, more complex cervical problems—such as whether your cervical mucus and your partner's sperm interact well together—require more precise testing. For now, though, unless you know there might be a problem, you can probably rest easy, knowing that there's only about a 5% chance that your cervix is hindering fertilization.

Uterine Factors

Once a doctor knows that a woman's ovaries are producing eggs, that her fallopian tubes are open, and that her cervix is not preventing sperm from entering, there is just one last factor left to evaluate: her uterus. For a pregnancy to be successful, the uterus must be up to its job of housing the developing fetus until it is ready to be born.

Uterine problems are fairly rare, though, and are a factor in infertility only about 5% of the time. Factors that can interfere with the uterus's ability to do its job include fibroids or endometrial scarring. If the uterus has an abnormal shape, then this, too, could lead to infertility.

You're at risk for having an abnormally shaped uterus if you were exposed to DES *in utero*—meaning that your mother took DES while she was pregnant with you. Typically, when DES is the culprit, the uterus is shaped like the letter "T" instead of an upside-down pear, which is what it should look like. As you can imagine, a T-shaped uterus isn't particularly adaptable to a fetus's growing shape. As a result, women with T-shaped uteruses are more inclined to have miscarriages or premature deliveries.

Besides DES exposure, other factors that can cause uterine abnormalities include previous D & Cs or abortions. These procedures can cause scar tissue and adhesions to form in the uterus, which, in turn, can alter the shape of the uterus and interfere with function. Other causes of uterine scar tissue include past IUD use, an infection, and sexually transmitted disease. Fibroids, or other benign growths called polyps, can also interfere with uterine function and cause miscarriages.

Without a thorough infertility workup, it can be difficult to know if you have a uterine abnormality. However, if you know you were exposed to DES while still in your mother's womb, then you know you have an increased risk for having a deformed uterus. Other than that, your only symptoms of a problem might be decreased menstrual bleeding if you have uterine scar tissue or adhesions, or increased or irregular menstrual bleeding if you have fibroids or polyps. Of course, these symptoms are less than specific because many factors can cause increased or decreased menstrual bleeding. Also, a misshapen uterus could produce no symptoms. The only way to know for sure whether or not your uterus is a problem is to undergo special testing that is part of an infertility evaluation.

But, even if you do have some type of a uterine disorder, this doesn't mean that you'll have to abandon your hopes for motherhood. Plenty of women with abnormally shaped uteruses, uterine scarring, or fibroids have become pregnant and carried their babies to term. However, a uterine abnormality would certainly increase your risk for being infertile.

Male Factors

Of course, the burden of becoming pregnant doesn't rest entirely on your shoulders. The man has a responsibility here, too. A man must be able to produce a sufficient number of good-quality sperm, and then be able to deliver those sperm into a woman's vagina, if fertilization is to occur. Although the male hormonal reproductive cycle is less complex than a woman's, there is still room for error.

For example, a man may have some defect that prevents him from producing enough sperm. This may result because of some genetic abnormality or may simply result because he's been exposed to high temperatures or environmental toxins. It may also result if, when he was born, one of his testicles remained stuck in his abdomen instead of having descended into his scrotum. This type of abnormality, when it occurs, is usually repaired at an early age. Regardless of when the surgery was performed, though, the quality of his semen will most likely be somewhat poor.[5] Other factors that can result in a poor sperm count include the presence of diabetes, a hormonal dysfunction, a varicocele, radiation therapy, and certain drugs. For example, anabolic steroids, taken by some athletes and bodybuilders to enhance muscle growth, drastically interfere with sperm production. Other drugs that can affect fertility include recreational drugs, such as narcotics and marijuana, as well as some prescription drugs, such as drugs taken to combat high blood pressure and depression.

Another factor that can affect a man's fertility is if his mother took DES while she was pregnant with him. Although the daughters of mothers who took DES have received most of the attention, the drug affected male infants as well. Researchers have found that men who were exposed to the drug *in utero* have an increased risk for having a poor semen analysis, and also for having cysts in the epididymis. As you may recall, the epididymis houses the sperm until they mature and are ready to leave the body in search of an egg. Cysts could interfere with the normal process of sperm maturation and delivery.

A man may also have a disorder that keeps the sperm from being deposited in the vagina. For example, the ducts that transport the sperm might be obstructed or deformed. He may also have a problem delivering sperm into the vagina because of factors ranging from poor technique to the fact that the ejaculate may exit into the bladder instead of out of the urethra (retrograde ejaculation).

For the most part, men who are infertile have no outward symptoms. About the only exception is in the case of retrograde ejaculation. In that disorder, a man experiences orgasm but no ejaculate comes out. Later, when he urinates, his urine is white with semen because the semen has entered his bladder instead of exiting his body.

This is the exception rather than the rule, though. Most men don't have any idea that they're infertile. The only way to know if a man is producing enough sperm is to have a sperm count performed. Actually, it's not a bad idea to have a sperm count run fairly early during the time you're attempting pregnancy. The test is simple and relatively inexpensive—at least as opposed to the more complex and often invasive tests performed on a woman's reproductive system—and its results could keep you from wasting valuable time and expending needless emotional energy worrying about why you haven't become pregnant.

*   *   *

Obvious signs of a fertility problem only occur in a fraction of the couples who have difficulty conceiving. Most have no signs or symptoms at all. The majority of women only know that, despite their best efforts to conceive, they continue to get their periods, same as always.

If you don't have any obvious sign of a fertility problem, and there's nothing in your history to suggest that you might be infertile, then when to seek help has to be left up to you. A basic guideline, though, is that whenever you feel there might be a problem, you should go ahead and consult an expert.

Choosing Your Doctor

Unfortunately, making the decision to consult an expert could be the easy part. Finding the best doctor for you can be more difficult.

Perhaps the most important thing you need to realize here is that just because a doctor calls himself an infertility specialist doesn't mean he is one. A doctor can have the word "INFERTILITY" on his door in big letters, but he still may not have any postgraduate training in this most precise field. And to make matters even more difficult for the consumer, increasing numbers of doctors are doing just that.

There are several reasons for this. One is simply the amount of money to be made in the field. As was discussed earlier, more and more couples are seeking infertility services, mainly because they have postponed childbearing and have a limited time in which to conceive. Another factor that motivates doctors to try to grab a piece of the infertility market relates to the costs of malpractice insurance. Obstetricians have one of the highest malpractice insurance rates in the business. On the other hand, an infertility practice has a much lower malpractice insurance rate. One reason for this is that, unlike with obstetrics, it's difficult to prove negligence. After all, even when treated appropriately, half of the couples seeking infertility treatment are ultimately unsuccessful. As you can see, this would make it very difficult to prove that a patient suffered an adverse outcome as a result of substandard care. So, for these reasons—increased income with decreased malpractice insurance rates—many doctors have decided to drop obstetrics from their practices and fill up the extra appointment slots with infertility patients.

That's why, when choosing a doctor, you can't let your guard down. You are the consumer. You are the one who wants a baby. So, as tempting as it may be just to turn everything over to an "expert" to "fix," don't. You need to be confident that the professional you are dealing with is truly an expert.

To make sure you will receive the best care possible, don't base your choice of a doctor solely on the recommendations of your friends. It's possible that your friends can provide some valuable names, that's true. But too many people draw a conclusion about a doctor's expertise because of his or her bedside manner. While feeling comfortable with a doctor is an important part of any medical workup, it certainly isn't the main thing. You need a doctor who knows what he's doing, who is an expert in the field of infertility. Many women have received treatment from doctors they thought were experts, only to find out, perhaps years and thousands of dollars later, that the doctors either didn't perform key tests or prescribed ineffective treatment.

So, feel free to ask around among your friends for the names of good doctors, but just don't take their recommendations as gospel. You'll also want to search out other names on your own. One way to do this is by looking in the yellow pages of the telephone book under the main heading "Physicians and Surgeons," and the subheadings "Infertility" or "Reproductive Endocrinology." You can also contact the American Fertility Society (2140 Eleventh Avenue South, Suite 200, Birmingham, Alabama 35205-2800; telephone number 205–933–8494) for the names of doctors in your area who specialize in infertility.

Another resource for the names of doctors specializing in infertility is a support group called Resolve. Resolve, which is based in Boston, Massachusetts, is a national support group for couples having problems with infertility. As a service to members, local chapters of Resolve keep lists of infertility specialists practicing in that area. All of the doctors whose names appear on this list have undergone a special evaluation process, which examines the doctor's experience along with his credentials. To find out more information about this service, contact your local chapter of Resolve. They are usually listed in the telephone book. If your town doesn't have a local chapter, contact the national headquarters at 1310 Broadway, Somerville, Massachusetts 02144-1731. Their phone number is (617) 643-0744.

Another way to learn more about the infertility specialists in your area is to find out the names of local hospitals that treat infertility patients. Then call the hospital and ask to speak to a nurse—preferably the head nurse—on the floor where most of these women stay when they're patients. Nurses can be a great source for information concerning various doctors. They work directly with a number of doctors, so they have a chance to learn, firsthand, how one doctor may compare to another. If you tell the nurse why you're seeking the information—that you're having difficulty becoming pregnant, that you're of an advanced age, that you have a minimum amount of time to lose, and you need to consult the best doctor possible—she will most likely be frank with her information and advice.

Once you have a list of doctors' names, call each doctor's office and try to gain as much information as you can over the telephone. Ask to speak to the doctor's nurse, and then briefly explain your situation. Tell her you're interested in becoming a patient but would like to ask a few questions first. Ask about the doctor's training and his credentials. For example, is he a board-certified reproductive endocrinologist, or is he an obstetrician/gynecologist who also treats infertility patients? (A reproductive endocrinologist has received specialized training in the area of reproductive medicine.) Next, ask how many patients the doctor sees a day for infertility problems, and what percentage of his practice constitutes infertility. (It's best if at least 50%, and preferably 85%, of the doctor's practice is infertility. After all, you want a doctor whose attention is focused on the causes of infertility.) Next, you may want to ask if the doctor delivers babies. If not, this could be a good sign; this would mean that the doctor most likely spends all of his time, and his energy, treating infertility.

Don't be swayed, though, by the fact that the doctor may be a member of the American Fertility Society or the Society of Assisted Reproductive Technology. Membership in one of these societies means that the doctor has an interest in infertility; it doesn't mean that he's an expert in the field. Both of these organizations have an open membership policy, meaning that any doctor can join, regardless of his credentials or his ethics. These societies maintain that their purpose is to provide doctors with educational material, not to evaluate a doctor's performance.

The information you receive in your telephone interview with the doctor's office should help you narrow your list to the doctors who seem the most promising. Your next step would then be to make an appointment to meet with these doctors personally. Although this is a preliminary interview, you need to be prepared to pay for the doctor's time. A one-hour consultation will most likely cost $150 or more. But this cost is miniscule compared to the cost of an infertility workup, and compared to your desire to have a child.

It's best if you and your partner can go to this first visit together. This is a joint undertaking, and a joint problem. Although many people think that infertility is primarily a female problem, this isn't true. In fact, the cause of a couple's infertility can be traced to the man about 35% of the time, to the woman about 35% of the time, and to both partners about 20% of the time. In the remaining 10%, no cause is ever found.[6] But, regardless of whose "fault" it is, the two of you should be in this together. After all, infertility is a *couple's* problem, not a problem to be assigned to one or the other partner.

When you finally meet the doctor, you'll want to ask how long he's specialized in infertility. Of course, the longer he's been practicing infertility, the more experienced he'll be. Ask him about the laboratory he works with, and whether the laboratory specializes in infertility. Again, you'll want a lab that is used to performing the precise tests that are part of an infertility workup. Next, ask about the hospital where the doctor admits patients. Is the hospital equipped to handle, and are the staff experienced in meeting, an infertility patient's specific needs? You may also want to ask the doctor whether or not he is qualified to perform tubal reconstructive surgery and if he performs *in vitro* fertilization or the GIFT (gamete intrafallopian transfer) procedure. If he does, you'll want to ask how many times he's performed the procedure, and what his success rate is.

Finally, you'll want to ask the doctor about how he would treat you if he were your doctor. He should have a definite, step-by-step plan. He should let you know when the tests should be completed and what he can learn from the tests. (The next chapter outlines in detail which tests should be performed and why.) If the doctor's approach appears haphazard or incomplete, then this isn't the doctor for you. The same thing goes if the doctor is impatient with answering your questions, or if he hurries you through your visit. An infertility workup, and any resultant treatment, can be lengthy and emotionally draining. You need a doctor who is thorough and who wants to make sure that you understand the purpose behind each test or recommendation.

Once you and your spouse have talked with the doctor, you

may want to think about what you've heard. If so, don't feel that you have to commit to this doctor for the complete workup. Simply thank him for his time, ask for any written information that you can review at home, and let him know that you'll think about what you've discussed. Remember: you're paying for the doctor's time. It's your decision as to whether you want him for a doctor, not his decision as to whether he wants you for a patient. But, if you feel comfortable with what the doctor has said, and you like his manner and approach, you may want to go ahead and tell the doctor that you're ready to become a patient. If that's the case, the doctor can proceed—most likely at this visit—with a medical history and a physical examination.

Many of the questions the doctor will ask during the medical history will seem quite personal. For example, the doctor will ask you about your menstrual history, whether or not you've had an abortion, how many different sexual partners you've had, and how frequently you currently have sex. But, although these questions are personal, they're necessary. The age at which you started menstruating is a clue as to whether your cycles are ovulatory. Whether or not you've had an abortion reveals that you were, at one time, able to conceive, but also shows that your uterus or cervix may have been damaged during the procedure. The number of sexual partners you've had, and the age at which you first had intercourse, says something about your risk for having had a pelvic infection. And, of course, how frequently you have sex may help explain why you haven't gotten pregnant. After taking a medical history, the doctor will perform a physical examination. Again, this first visit should take about an hour. If it doesn't—for example, say that it only takes ten or fifteen minutes—then this isn't the right doctor for you.

Throughout this entire process, don't ever feel "locked in" to one particular doctor. Never forget that you are paying for the doctor's time, and you have the right to know what to expect. Don't feel intimidated or pressured into consenting to treatment when you don't feel comfortable doing so. At the same time, if you begin treatment with one doctor, and you feel like something's not being done the way it should, feel free to get either a second opinion or switch doctors. Some people begin to cave in a little here. They may tell themselves, "He's done so much already. His feelings will be hurt if I switch." That's nonsense. You are paying for a service. Although your doctor no doubt cares about your best interests, he is, at heart, a businessman. Medicine is his business, and you are paying his salary. Never hesitate to ask for your records to get a second opinion if you want one. Any reputable physician would have absolutely no complaint about your doing so; in fact, he'd probably encourage it.

To illustrate exactly how big of a business infertility treatments are, consider this: according to the Office of Technology Assessment, infertile couples in the United States spent about $1 billion in 1987 on medical treatments aimed at conception.[7] Furthermore, between 1965 and 1982, the number of infertility-related visits to a physician rose from 600,000 each year to 1.6 million; however, the number of infertile couples remained about the same.[8] This can only mean that doctors are performing more tests, and administering more treatments, to infertile couples today than ever before. Some of these tests and treatments are warranted; some aren't. Often it will be left up to you to differentiate between the two. You can do this through research, so you know what to expect, and through obtaining second opinions. This is a lot of work, there's no question. But hopefully the payoff will be worth it.

Conclusion

Not everyone needs to consult a doctor because of problems becoming pregnant. Some women get pregnant without any difficulty at all. However, many, many others *do* have difficulty and do end up seeking medical help. This is especially true when age is an issue.

If you end up consulting a doctor, you can feel confident that you're one step ahead of the process. You now know the basics about the types of things that could be disrupting your plans for pregnancy. You also know the qualities and credentials to look for when choosing a doctor to help you through this sometimes difficult process of conception.

But, keep in mind that, even after you've selected a doctor, you need to remain on top of the evaluation process. Even the best doctors can get busy and forget things. By becoming familiar with the tests that are part of a basic infertility evaluation, you can be sure that you're doing everything necessary to help you achieve your goal of parenthood.

8

The Evaluation Process

If the time comes when you find yourself facing a workup for infertility, you need to know what to expect. The process is intensive, but, after just two to three months, an infertility specialist should, in most instances, be able to identify why you've been having difficulty conceiving. Of course, that's assuming you've selected an accomplished specialist, one who will correctly perform all of the tests necessary. That's why this chapter is so important. By knowing, in advance, exactly what's involved in a workup, not only will you be prepared for the time and money you'll have to spend, you'll also be assured of receiving an evaluation that is both complete and appropriate.

The Complete Workup

An infertility workup should follow a definite, organized plan, with every test having a specific function. Basically, an infertility workup will evaluate whether your ovaries are operational, your fallopian tubes are open, your cervix is functioning, and your uterus is normal. It will also evaluate whether your partner is producing enough sperm. It's possible to complete the entire battery of tests in as little as two or three months. Of course, that means having to undergo several tests during any one month. That's intensive, to be sure. But, when you're through with all the tests, you'll have a better picture of your reproductive health and, hopefully, be on your way to solving any problem. Even when no cause for the infertility can be found—which happens in about 10% of the cases—the doctor can still use the information furnished by the tests to recommend ways to help facilitate a pregnancy.

The key here, though, is that you follow through with all of the tests. Each test evaluates just one aspect of your reproductive ability, so stopping after a less-than-complete workup will give you a less-than-complete idea of what's going on in your reproductive organs. Even if an early test uncovers a specific problem, you still need to continue on and finish the rest of the tests. One reason for this is that, in many cases, infertility has more than one cause. For example, let's say that your doctor discovers that you're not ovulating regularly. "Ah ha," you both say, "that's what the problem's been." Confident that you've finally found the answer, you start taking medication to stimulate ovulation. But, the months drag on and you're still not pregnant. Your doctor then decides to complete the infertility testing. After a few more tests, you and your doctor discover that your fallopian tubes are blocked. Think how devastating that would be: all of those months taking medications to make yourself ovulate, and the ovum didn't have a way to get to the uterus.

Another reason to complete testing before beginning any treatment is that some treatments, particularly medications, can interfere with the results of certain tests. For example, a commonly prescribed fertility drug, called clomiphene (often known by the trade name Clomid), can interfere with endometrial development or impair the quality of cervical mucus. Let's say you start taking clomiphene before you've completed the basic workup. After many months, you're still not pregnant so the doctor performs a test that revealing that you're not producing enough cervical mucus. Now you're stuck in the predicament of not knowing whether that's been a problem all along, or whether that's simply a side effect of the clomiphene.

The obvious solution to both of these problems is to complete the entire workup before beginning any treatment. That's the only way to have a full, accurate picture of your reproductive health.

The Cost of a Workup

As you can well imagine, the cost of a complete workup varies, depending upon where you live and even whom you consult. But, on average, a complete, basic workup (including a laparoscopy) will run between $4000 and $6000. How much of this will be covered by insurance depends upon your specific policy. Some policies won't pay for any part of an infertility workup, maintaining that such testing is "elective" and that your health doesn't depend upon your being able to have a baby. But, while an insurance company may deny coverage for a procedure that has the sole purpose of diagnosing infertility, it will pay if the doctor can show that the procedure is necessary for your overall health. For example, one part of an infertility workup is a laparoscopy, a surgical procedure that allows the doctor to examine your reproductive organs. If the sole reason for the laparoscopy is to diagnose infertility, an insurance company may deny coverage. But, if the doctor can show that he's also using the procedure to identify the source of pelvic pain or to rule out endometriosis—both conditions that could endanger a woman's health—then the insurance company would most likely pay for the procedure.

To know for sure what your policy does or does not cover, contact your insurance company representative. One tip: if your insurance policy doesn't specifically exclude infertility treatments, it may be possible for you to force them to cover your care even if they later try to deny coverage. Of course, this probably won't be easy. You'd have to be persistent, calling and writing letters to those in upper management positions. But the time and effort may very well pay off. Another option is to discuss the situation with your doctor; he might have some ideas of his own as to how your workup can be covered by insurance.

Basic Infertility Tests

Regardless of where you live, or whom you consult, a basic infertility evaluation should contain, in addition to a thorough history and physical examination, certain key tests. These tests are designed to determine what factor, or factors, might be interfering with your ability to conceive. The causative factor might be related to your ovaries, fallopian tubes, cervix, uterus, or your partner's sperm. To ensure that you are receiving the evaluation you need, make sure that your workup contains all of the following tests.

Evaluation of the Ovaries

It stands to reason that a major part of any infertility evaluation involves making sure that ovulation is occurring. Your doctor will most likely gain evidence of ovulation by evaluating your basal body temperature chart, which was discussed in detail in Chapter 6, and by analyzing the hormones in your blood and your endometrial lining. In certain instances, the doctor may want to use an ultrasound to confirm that ovulation is indeed occurring.

Blood Hormone Testing

Hormone levels change each and every day of a menstrual cycle. Follicle stimulating hormone, or FSH, rises in the beginning of a cycle to encourage an egg to mature. About this same time, the hormone estrogen also enters your bloodstream, which motivates the uterus to develop its endometrial lining and encourages the cervix to produce mucus. Then, about midcycle, the hormone LH surges, causing a mature egg to break free from the ovary. The site that remains after ovulation—the corpus luteum—then begins to secrete the hormone progesterone. Progesterone sees to it that the uterus holds onto its endometrial lining until all concerned are certain that conception hasn't occurred.

It's by testing the level of the hormone progesterone during the last half of your menstrual cycle that the doctor can gain some clue as to whether or not ovulation has occurred. It only stands to reason: if you don't ovulate, you won't have a corpus luteum; if you don't have a corpus luteum, your level of progesterone will be low. Or, even if you do ovulate, your level of progesterone could still be low if your corpus luteum isn't producing the amount of progesterone the uterine lining needs to maintain itself. Performing a blood test to check your level of progesterone will cost about $50.

A serum progesterone level of at least 3 to 4 ng/ml three to four days before your period is due to start suggests that you did, indeed, ovulate.[1] Be aware, though, that the corpus luteum doesn't secrete progesterone in a constant, steady stream. Instead, it produces progesterone in small bursts. Therefore, the level of progesterone in your blood on any given morning may very well be different than the level in your blood the next day, or even that same afternoon. In fact, some studies suggest that morning progesterone levels tend to be consistently higher than those drawn in the evening. Because of these variable results, many doctors feel that the basal body temperature chart and endometrial biopsy, which is discussed later in this section, add important information to help confirm that ovulation is proceeding normally.

Other hormones you may wish to ask your doctor about checking—especially if you've delayed childbearing until an age when you feel you might be approaching menopause—are FSH, LH, and estrogen. Although there is no definite test that will tell you whether your reproductive organs are feeling the effects of age, the levels of these hormones just might give some clue. Researchers have found that, for a few years preceding menopause, the hormone FSH rises more than usual in the first half of the cycle while the hormone estrogen, or estradiol, rises less. At the same time, the blood level of progesterone may be normal.[2] Therefore, if you were to rely solely on progesterone levels for information about your reproductive health, you could conclude that you're ovulating normally. But, if the hormones FSH and estrogen are out of whack, you may not be ovulating normally, after all.

Furthermore, if your temperature chart shows that you ovulate before midcycle—meaning that you have a shortened follicular phase, the phase when the ovum matures—then your blood levels of FSH, LH, and estrogen may be especially revealing. In this instance, if you have an increased level of FSH and a normal level of LH early in your cycle, then you could very well be approaching menopause.[3] And if this is the case, you could have a very hard time becoming pregnant, either on your own or with medical help.

You need to know, though, that there is no absolute test for whether or not a woman is approaching menopause. These tests—which cost about $50 each—are simply indicators. Keep in mind, too, that the hormones FSH and LH vary significantly each and every day of the cycle. This means that it can be difficult to draw any conclusion about the effects of age, or about the state of the ovaries, based on these tests alone.[4] Even so, the hormone FSH is the most sensitive marker available to help a woman know whether or not she is approaching menopause.[5]

Other hormone levels that may be checked, especially if your doctor suspects that you have a problem with ovulation, include prolactin and thyroid. Even slight abnormalities in either of these hormones can disrupt ovulation. Blood tests for both prolactin and thyroid hormone cost about $40 each. Also, if you have any signs of excess male hormone production—such as excess hair growth on your face, oily skin, acne, or thinning of the hair on your head—then the doctor will want to run a blood test to check for excess androgen production. Besides disrupting ovulation, an elevated level of androgens could also signal a more serious problem, such as an ovarian tumor.

Endometrial Biopsy

Even more reliable than checking the level of progesterone in your blood is checking to see if the progesterone that's being produced by the corpus luteum is doing its job; and, as you already know, its job is to develop and maintain the endometrium. Actually, the endometrium has two stages of growth. The first stage occurs during the first half of the menstrual cycle, when estrogen stimulates the cells of the endometrium to begin to proliferate. The second stage occurs just after ovulation, when the corpus luteum begins pumping progesterone into your system. This sudden infusion of progesterone causes the endometrial cells to change in a very predictable manner. The changes are so predictable, in fact, that by simply analyzing a small sample of endometrial tissue, a trained technician can state how many days previously ovulation occurred. This fact can tell the doctor two things.

First, it can help confirm whether or not ovulation occurred. For example, if the sample shows that it hasn't been influenced by progesterone at all, then it's probably safe to conclude that progesterone wasn't available, which would mean that ovulation didn't occur. After all: no ovulation, no corpus luteum; no corpus luteum, no progesterone.

Second, it can reveal whether the endometrium is maturing normally. As you may well imagine, if the endometrium lags behind in its development, and a fertilized egg arrives, then the endometrium may not be ready to meet the growing egg's needs. As a result, the egg would slough off.

This condition, called a luteal phase inadequacy, occurs either because the corpus luteum is weak and simply can't produce enough progesterone to satisfy the endometrium, or because the corpus luteum peaks too soon in progesterone production, causing the levels of the hormone to taper off at a time when they should remain stable. It's also possible that the endometrium, for some reason, can't respond to the progesterone that the corpus luteum is making available.[6] Regardless, a blood test alone won't reveal a luteal phase inadequacy. It's possible to have a normal level of progesterone in the blood and still have abnormal endometrial development. That's why an endometrial biopsy may be necessary.

The biopsy should be performed as close to the first day of menstruation as possible, but before bleeding actually begins. Therefore, if you usually menstruate every 28 days, you'll want to schedule the biopsy about day 26 or day 27 of your cycle. Performed in the doctor's office, the test doesn't require any advance preparation. You'll lie down on the examining table and place your feet in the stirrups, just as you would for a pelvic exam. After inserting a speculum, the doctor will slide a very thin, flexible tube through your vagina and into your uterine cavity. He'll then either scrape the tube along the side of your uterus or use a suction device to obtain a bit of tissue. You'll probably feel some cramping as the doctor does this, but rest assured that the pain will be short-lived. You may also experience some spotting after the test is completed.

Once the doctor has obtained the sample of tissue, he'll send it to a laboratory for analysis. The laboratory will then date the tissue according to its characteristics. For example, if the tissue appears to have the same characteristics as an endometrium that has been developing for 12 days after ovulation has occurred, then the pathologist will date it as being postovulatory day 12, or day 26. (For the sake of the test, the pathologist assumes that ovulation occurred on day 14; therefore, 14 plus 12 equals 26.) This number in itself, though, has no relevance. To find out if the tissue is normal, the doctor must then compare the date assigned to the tissue to the date of your actual cycle, which means counting backwards from the date your *next* period begins. The day your period starts automatically becomes day 28, regardless of how many days previously your last period began. So, if your period starts two days after you've had the biopsy, then that day will become day 28. You'll then count backwards to the day the biopsy was taken. In this case, it was two days before, so, in effect, the biopsy was taken on day 26 of your cycle. This is the same date assigned to the endometrium by the pathologist, which means that the endometrium is normal, or "in phase."

On the other hand, if the pathologist felt that the endometrial tissue only reflected eight days' development after ovulation, he would have dated it day 22. In this case, there would be a four-day discrepancy between the date the biopsy was actually taken and the date assigned by the pathologist. This would mean that the endometrium was lagging behind in its development by about four days, which would constitute a luteal phase inadequacy. Most experts feel that a two- to three-day, or greater, discrepancy between the actual cycle date and the date assigned to the endometrium by the pathologist constitutes a luteal phase inadequacy.

Now, the significance of this information is another matter altogether. For one thing, some normal, fertile women can occasionally have a cycle with an inadequate luteal phase. For this reason, most experts feel that, to definitively diagnose the problem, biopsies must be taken during different cycles to make sure that the problem is consistently occurring. Furthermore, even after it's diagnosed, it's not at all clear as to how significant a problem a luteal phase inadequacy really is. In fact, some experts aren't sure whether luteal phase inadequacy is a significant factor in causing infertility; they also aren't sure that treating it will make any difference in whether or not a woman will become pregnant.[7,8] (Luteal phase inadequacy may, however, be a factor in causing recurrent miscarriages.) In addition, luteal phase inadequacy is relatively rare; it affects only 3 to 4% of all infertile women.[9] For these reasons, you may wish to question your doctor as to whether or not this test is absolutely necessary.

All in all, an endometrial biopsy may help to give a better overall view of your menstrual cycle; it also may help predict whether or not you'll have a problem with miscarriages. At times, too, a luteal phase inadequacy may be the only abnormality found, meaning that this may be the only information on which your doctor has to base treatment recommendations. For these reasons, your doctor may wish to run the test and you may wish to go along with it. If you do have the test, be assured that the test is safe and simple. But, because the test is performed during the last half of a menstrual cycle, there is a chance—although a very slight chance—that the test could disturb an embryo and cause a miscarriage if you just happened to be pregnant that cycle. For this reason, most doctors will run a pregnancy test before performing the biopsy—just in case. The endometrial biopsy alone costs about $90.

Ultrasound

All of the tests mentioned so far can only suggest that ovulation has occurred. A test that can help underscore those findings is an ultrasound of the ovaries. Performed in the doctor's office, an ultrasound uses sound waves to create an image of the ovaries on a televisionlike screen. The doctor can then watch the development of follicles, which look like blisters, on the ovaries; these follicles contain eggs that are maturing in preparation for ovulation. Over successive days, at least one follicle will grow larger and larger. Then, on the day of ovulation, the follicle will appear dramatically smaller on ultrasound, meaning that the egg has broken free. Also, if the doctor can spy a small puddle of fluid at the bottom of the peritoneal cavity behind the uterus, then this is further evidence that ovulation has occurred; this fluid is what drains out of the follicle when the egg finally breaks free.

The ultrasound is easy to perform, and it's safe. It doesn't harm the eggs because no radiation is being used. To have an ultrasound, you'd lie on an examining table while a technician or your doctor inserts a long, thin object that looks like a microphone (called a transducer) into your vagina. The technician would then watch the monitor screen as the transducer transmitted images of your internal organs. By moving the transducer around, he'd be able to create a picture of both your right and left ovaries.

An ultrasound is painless and only takes a few minutes to perform. The test has its drawbacks, though. For one thing, unless you'd timed your LH surge precisely, you could miss seeing the collapse of the follicle and conclude that you didn't ovulate when, in fact, you did. For example, sometimes a follicle that has released an egg will reseal and again fill with fluid. So, if you were just a day or so late with the ultrasound, you could see this refilled follicle and wrongly think that the follicle never released an egg.

Another drawback is the cost. Just one ultrasound can cost from $60 to $150. To detect ovulation, you'd need to have a series of ultrasounds—at least three or so—performed. As you can see, at $150 a pop, this could add up in a hurry.

Evaluation of the Uterus and Fallopian Tubes

Properly functioning fallopian tubes are integral to the process of conception. As we've discussed previously, not only must the fallopian tube reach up to catch an ovulating egg, it must work to propel an egg down the tube while it's simultaneously encouraging sperm to make their way up the tube. Unfortunately, though, the testing that's available can only evaluate whether the tubes are open, or patent—the tests can't show whether the tubes are otherwise functioning. Of course, if the tube isn't open, this would be a major stumbling block to any attempts at conception.

The most commonly used test to evaluate whether the fallopian tubes are open and able to act as passageways is an X-ray test called the hysterosalpingogram. The name of this test may seem unpronounceable; but, when you break the word down, not only is it pronounceable, it also makes sense. "Hystero" (as in "hysterectomy") means uterus; "salpingo" (with a hard "g") means fallopian tubes; "gram" refers to an examination of. Therefore, hysterosalpingogram is simply an X-ray of the uterus and fallopian tubes. In this instance, the test requires the injection of dye through the cervix and into the uterine cavity to make the uterus and fallopian tubes visible on X-ray.

The best time to have the test performed is in the first half of the menstrual cycle, after you've stopped bleeding but before you've ovulated. There are two reasons for this timing. First, if you were still bleeding from your period, it's possible that the injection of dye into the uterus could propel the sloughing endometrial tissue up through your uterus, out the ends of your fallopian tubes, and into your peritoneal cavity. Once the endometrial tissue landed in your peritoneal cavity, it's possible, at least theoretically, for the errant tissue to develop into endometriosis. The second reason for having the test performed in the first half of the cycle is so the injection of the dye doesn't accidentally disrupt a pregnancy. Again, it's possible that the force of the dye could push a fertilized egg out your fallopian tube and into your peritoneal cavity, causing an ectopic pregnancy.[10]

To prepare for the test, it's a good idea to begin taking an antibiotic—usually doxycycline—for two days before the test and then to continue taking the medication for three days after the test. The reason for this is that the injection of dye could cause any latent infection to rage out of control. It would be tragic, indeed, to develop an infection in your fallopian tubes because of a test that is designed to help diagnose fertility problems, especially when simply taking an antibiotic could prevent this from happening.[11]

To have the test performed, you'd most likely go to an X-ray facility, or you might have it performed in a hospital as an outpatient. You would then lie on an examining table with your feet in stirrups, just as you would before a pelvic examination. After inserting a speculum and cleansing your vagina, the radiologist or your doctor would inject dye into your uterus while taking X-rays. The dye should flow through your uterus—outlining the shape of the uterus and revealing any fibroids or polyps—and up into your fallopian tubes. If your fallopian tubes are open, the dye will flow out of the tubes and into your peritoneal cavity. But, if your tubes are blocked, the dye will stop, or at least narrow, at the site of the blockage. Then, by carefully watching how the dye accumulates in the peritoneal cavity, the doctor may discern whether any scar tissue or adhesions are lurking in the vicinity of your reproductive organs.

The test only takes about 10 to 20 minutes to perform, but— be forewarned—it does cause brief cramping. Taking one or two 200 mg tablets of ibuprofen (Advil, Motrin, Nuprin) an hour or two before the test may help relieve the discomfort. The test costs about $500 to $600. Yes, that's expensive and, yes, the test is uncomfortable. But, the information gleaned from the exam can be valuable.

For example, a hysterosalpingogram can identify whether your uterus is shaped normally, and whether it contains fibroids or polyps, which could interfere with a pregnancy. Even more important, it can reveal whether your fallopian tubes are open and ready to receive an egg. But the test is limited. For one thing, the X-ray doesn't give any information about the *outside* of these organs. Scar tissue from endometriosis could be pinning your fallopian tubes in place, preventing them from assuming the positions necessary for optimum fertility, and yet, the hysterosalpingogram could look completely normal. On the other hand, the sudden rush of dye can, at times, cause the fallopian tubes to spasm, cutting off the flow of dye and giving the false impression of a blockage.

Despite these shortcomings, the hysterosalpingogram is still a useful test. Short of surgery, there's nothing else that can tell you as much about the state of these vital, but hidden, reproductive organs.

Evaluation of the Cervix

The next structure to come under scrutiny is the cervix. We've already discussed how important the cervix is in the process of fertilization. The cervix must, around the time of ovulation, produce enough nourishing, hospitable mucus so that sperm want to enter and linger for a few days. As you may recall, the cervix acts as a way station, a place where sperm can congregate and live for several days; with such hospitable surroundings, the sperm can then break free at their leisure, darting forth in search of a ripe egg. If not for the cervix, the sperm would die in a matter of hours instead of days, greatly diminishing the chances for conception.

To determine whether your cervix is helping or hindering your desires for pregnancy, your doctor will want to perform a postcoital test. This test involves an examination of your cervical mucus around the time of ovulation after you and your partner have had sexual intercourse. The postcoital test reveals a couple of things. First, it will show whether your cervix is producing the abundant, clear mucus it should be at that point in your cycle. Second, it will reveal whether your partner's sperm are able to survive in your cervical mucus.

The timing for this test is critical. Cervical mucus is at its optimum for the brief period immediately before ovulation. So, you need to schedule the test for a time before, but as close as possible to, the day you expect to ovulate. This means that if you normally ovulate on day 14 of your cycle, the test should be performed on day 12 or 13. To make sure the test is timed appropriately, either use an ovulation predictor kit to detect your LH surge, or keep a temperature chart for the month in which the test is performed. Although the temperature chart won't alert you to impending ovulation, it may help confirm after the fact whether or not the test was performed on the correct day. That could be important if the quality or quantity of your cervical mucus is at all borderline. Being late by just a day or two can make a world of difference in the results of the test; as soon as ovulation occurs, the cervical mucus changes consistency and begins to dry up.

If your cycle is irregular, timing the postcoital test could be difficult. If worse comes to worse, the doctor may need to regulate your cycle through the use of a medication, such as clomiphene, before performing the test.

Timing is the most difficult part of the postcoital test; the rest is easy. To perform the test, you and your partner would have sexual intercourse after having abstained for a couple of days. You should avoid using any lubricants or douches, and, after intercourse, remain lying in bed for about 30 minutes to give the sperm a head start on their trip into the cervix. Then, after waiting a certain period of time, you would go to your doctor's office for a pelvic examination. Exactly how long you'd need to wait between having sex and showing up at your doctor's office will depend on the doctor. Many doctors instruct their patients to come in two to three hours after intercourse. Others feel that waiting about 10 hours is better. For one thing, this delayed timing makes it easier on the patient's schedule by allowing them to have sex the night before a morning appointment, or the morning before an afternoon visit. In addition, it helps give a more accurate portrayal of the cervix's ability to act as a reservoir for the sperm.[12] After all, sperm should be able to survive in the cervix for at least 24 hours; if they're all dead after only 10 hours, then fertility may be decreased.

Once you arrive at the doctor's office, the doctor will perform a pelvic examination. The exam may seem like a routine pelvic exam, but the doctor will actually be looking for several things. First, he'll check to make sure the cervix is producing an abundance of clear mucus. If it's not, and the mucus available is on the skimpy side, then this could mean that a contingent of sperm may not be able to survive there very long. Next, the doctor will take a small bit of mucus and try to stretch it. If the mucus is very elastic, this will help confirm that the timing of the test is accurate and that ovulation is pending. To confirm his finding, he'll place another small sample of mucus on a microscope slide and allow it to dry. If ovulation is pending, the mucus should dry in a pattern that resembles the leaves of a fern.

Next, the doctor will take another sample of mucus, place it on a slide, and examine it under a microscope. He'll search the sample for active, moving sperm. Exactly how many sperm should be present is a matter of debate. As a guideline, the American Fertility Society says that a sample of cervical mucus taken from the center of the cervix about 10 hours after sexual intercourse should reveal about 10 motile sperm when examined under the high-power field of a microscope.[13] If fewer than 10 hours has elapsed since intercourse, even more sperm should be present.

Even more important than how many sperm are present is whether the sperm that are there are alive, swimming actively, and looking ready to break free and travel. If the sperm are dead, then one of three things are possible. First, they could have arrived that way, in which case a sperm analysis would also show dead sperm. Second, it could be that something in the cervical mucus—such as an infection or antibodies—killed them. Third, it could be that the test was performed at the wrong time.

Besides being dead, the sperm might be shaking in place and not making forward progress. Such aimless activity again raises a suspicion that antibodies in the cervical mucus are attacking and incapacitating the sperm.

If the results of the test are less than optimum, for whatever reason, the first thing to do is simply repeat the test. The most common cause of an abnormal postcoital test is poor timing. Remember: cervical mucus is in its prime for only a very brief period. Missing that prime time by just a day or two could drastically influence the test results. Also, if you waited more than two or three hours between having sex and receiving the evaluation, the doctor may want you to come in earlier for the repeat test. In some women, the sperm only survive in the cervical mucus for two to two and a half hours, but the women are still fertile.[14]

If you have a second postcoital test that's been carefully timed, and the test still shows sperm that are either dead or shaking in place, then something may be wrong, either with your cervical mucus or with the sperm themselves. Be reassured, though, that an abnormal postcoital test does not necessarily mean that you won't be able to conceive. Many couples have become pregnant after having several abnormal postcoital tests. But, at the same time, if you have an abnormal test, you'll want to try to identify the reason why if you can. The first step would be to make sure you don't have an infection in your cervix that's killing the sperm. If that's not the case, the next step may be to check to see if antibodies—which could be present either in your mucus or in your husband's semen—are attacking the sperm and causing them to die.

Antisperm Antibody Testing

The body produces antibodies—dozens of different kinds of antibodies—which are designed to attack foreign invaders, such as bacteria and viruses. Each particular antibody has been programmed to fight and kill one specific invader. For example, because you were immunized against diphtheria as a child, your body has antibodies designed specifically to ward off the diphtheria bacteria. But these same antibodies would be useless if confronted by a flu virus.

Although it rarely happens, it's possible for a man's or a woman's body to mistakenly identify sperm as foreign invaders and to manufacture antibodies against them. It's not clear why this occurs. But, when a man produces antibodies against his own sperm, the production of sperm usually suffers. When a woman produces antibodies against her partner's sperm, the sperm may be attacked and incapacitated the moment they enter the reproductive tract.

Because these antibodies are programmed to fight against sperm, they latch onto the sperm and then work to trip up the sperm on each leg of their journey. First, the antibodies may try to keep the sperm from entering the cervical mucus; if the sperm manage to enter the cervix anyway, the antibodies may make it difficult for them to survive there. Even if some of the sperm manage to escape the hostile environment of the cervix, anti-bodies may prevent them from fertilizing an egg.

Despite this neat little scenario, the whole issue of anti-sperm antibodies is wrought with controversy. One reason for the confusion is that it's possible for a man or woman to have antisperm antibodies and to have absolutely no problem becoming pregnant. However, there is a possibility—although it's a slight possibility—that antisperm antibodies could interfere with conception.

If your doctor feels you and your partner should be tested for antisperm antibodies, there are a few things of which you need to be aware. First, ask about the type of test that will be used to check for the antibodies. The reason for this is that some doctors—especially if they're not up-to-date on infertility tests—may simply order a blood test to check for the presence of antibodies. But, experts now know that just because a man or a woman has antisperm antibodies in his or her blood, there's no proof that the antibodies are interfering with fertility.[15] Further-more, a test for antisperm antibodies that is performed directly on sperm also doesn't have much clinical significance.

The one test that does have clinical significance is called immunobead binding. This type of test—which costs about $100—is much more sensitive than the other tests. By using this method to examine the blood of the man or the woman along with the sperm of the man, a technician can actually see which sperm have antibodies attached. Not only that, he can also tell *where* on the sperm the antibody has attached itself. Knowing how many sperm have antibodies, and where the antibodies are located, is crucial to making a determination as to whether or not the antibodies are interfering with fertility. For example, if most of the sperm are free of the unwanted antibodies, and if those sperm are otherwise healthy, then fertility probably isn't being impaired at all. Also, even if quite a number of the sperm have antibodies, but the antibodies are simply swinging along on the tail of the sperm, there's a good chance that those sperm could still penetrate an egg. Again, this would mean that the antibodies weren't interfering with fertility. But, if the antibody is smothering the head of the sperm, the sperm probably couldn't drill into an egg. In this instance, the antibodies could be interfering with the process of conception.

Okay, let's say that you have the antibody test and the results come back positive. What then? Unfortunately, there's no clear-cut answer. Many of the treatments doctors have used in the past, some of which some doctors still prescribe, may not help the problem. Not only that, some treatments may actually hinder your cause and hurt your health.

One tried but not-so-true treatment requires the partner of a woman with antisperm antibodies to wear a condom during intercourse. The theory is that, by decreasing the woman's exposure to the sperm, the woman's body will reduce its production of antibodies after a period of time. A major disadvantage here, obviously, is that your goal is to become pregnant, not to prevent conception. Other than that one rather obvious handicap, the treatment hasn't proved very successful in eliminating antibodies.[16]

Another treatment has required the person with the antibodies to take corticosteroid medications. Your body normally produces a certain amount of steroids to help you withstand stress. If a person supplements this supply with corticosteroid medication, one result is that the immune system becomes suppressed. Knowing this, doctors have reasoned that, by suppressing the immune system with corticosteroids, the production of antibodies would naturally decrease. Furthering this theory, some studies actually showed that steroids successfully decreased the number of antisperm antibodies; however, other studies showed no such effect.[17] Even more important than these equivocal results, though, is the fact that the treatment itself can harm your health. Corticosteroids are potent medications. Because your immune system is suppressed, you could be more susceptible to infection. Another serious side effect is aseptic necrosis of the hip, an irreversible condition where the hip joint decays and finally collapses.

Still other doctors have tried washing the sperm to remove the antibodies and then using artificial insemination to instill the cleansed sperm into the woman's uterus. However, the effectiveness of this therapy is also debatable. On the positive side, one group of researchers reported that they had achieved about a 40% pregnancy rate in women with antisperm antibodies after stimulating their ovaries with clomiphene and then artificially inseminating them with washed sperm.[18] In contrast, another study showed that one could wash sperm as many as 18 times without reducing the number of antibodies.[19]

Despite all of these dismal findings, being told you have antisperm antibodies doesn't mean you'll have to give up your plans for pregnancy. Some women get pregnant despite positive antibody tests. Even more encouraging, though, is that couples who have antisperm antibodies have been successful becoming pregnant with procedures such as *in vitro* fertilization and GIFT (which are discussed in detail in Chapter 9).[20]

Evaluation of the Male

Because so many of the infertility tests focus on the female, people often jump to the conclusion that the woman is the primary cause of a couple's fertility problem. But that's far from true. As has already been mentioned, the male is at least a contributor to, if not the sole factor in, a couple's infertility about 40% of the time. For this reason, your partner *must* receive a complete evaluation, including a semen analysis. In fact, because sperm counts vary, often dramatically, from month to month, he should have two to three tests performed over a two- to three-month period. A variety of factors can alter the results of a semen analysis, including stress, alcohol consumption, the frequency of ejaculation, and even the time of year. Scientists have found that, in most men, sperm counts follow a regular, annual rhythm, with the count reaching its highest values between February and March and dipping to an annual low in September.[21]

The semen analysis is a relatively simple test. Costing

somewhere between $50 and $90, there are no restrictions on when the test can be performed. The only prerequisite is that the man abstain from ejaculation for two to three days before the analysis to keep from having a falsely low sperm count. However, don't take this to mean that a man can significantly raise his motile sperm count by abstaining from sex for more than four or five days. Abstaining from sex for more than about seven to ten days could cause the sperm to begin to die. Therefore, although the total number of sperm in the ejaculate may increase slightly after abstaining from sex for an extended period, many of these sperm would be dead and incapable of fertilizing an egg.

When collecting a semen sample for analysis, the best method, by far, is masturbation. Some men may find this distasteful and perhaps even difficult. That's understandable, but they need to persevere. For the semen results to be accurate, the lab needs to have every drop of the ejaculate. That's why masturbation is the best method; no other method can collect the entire sample. Even the withdrawal technique, where a man withdraws his penis from the woman's vagina just before ejaculating, isn't adequate. No matter how disciplined a man is, he probably won't be able to withdraw in time to catch the very first drop of ejaculate; and it's that first drop that contains the highest concentration of sperm. So, if the first drop of ejaculate doesn't make it into the collection container, the odds are good that the sperm count will be falsely low. It's also not a good idea to use a condom to collect the sample. Besides the fact that most condoms contain a spermicide, which will kill the sperm, a portion of the sample will be lost, stuck to the sides of the condom. It is possible, though, to buy condoms that don't contain a spermicide. So, if your partner absolutely must use a technique other than masturbation, then a condom that doesn't contain a spermicide is the lesser of two evils.

It's also worth noting that the circumstances under which your partner collects his semen sample will affect the quality of the sample. For example, studies have shown that the quality of the semen improves if the man is sexually excited. Therefore, it's important that the man collect the sample in an environment in which he is comfortable—such as at home rather than in a bathroom at a clinic—and that he also use some means to help him become aroused.

Now that you know the best method for collecting the sample, into what do you put it? The best choice is a clean, glass jar with a wide mouth. The wide mouth makes collection easier, and glass seems to be less noxious to sperm than plastic. Your doctor's office should also be able to furnish you with a special container made out of plastic that's not toxic to sperm. Either way, it's a good idea to keep the jar small—say one to two ounces—so that the semen doesn't end up simply coating, and then drying along, the sides of the jar.

Once your partner has collected the sample, he needs to make sure that it arrives at the lab within an hour. Outside the cozy confines of the reproductive tract, the sperm begin to die; so, the sooner it's analyzed, the better. Also keep in mind that sperm like a nice, even temperature. Instruct whoever transports the specimen to keep it as close to body temperature as possible. This means placing the sample next to the body if the weather is cold.

Once the specimen arrives at the lab, the lab technicians will go to work. First, they'll check the sample for its consistency, or viscosity. Immediately after ejaculation, semen is thick and slightly gel-like in consistency, probably so that it won't leak out of the vagina immediately after intercourse. Within 5 to 20 minutes, though, the sample needs to liquefy so that the sperm can glide freely. If it doesn't, the extra-thick semen can trap the sperm, making it difficult for them to move. Semen that refuses to liquefy could result from an infection in the prostate or seminal vesicles, or it could simply occur for no known reason.

After checking the viscosity, the technician will measure the volume of the semen. Ideally, the volume should be between 2.5 and 8 ml, which is equivalent to about 1/2 to 1 teaspoon. Even if the volume is low, this doesn't necessarily mean that the sperm count is low. The volume of semen has nothing to do with the number of sperm that are available. However, sperm need a certain amount of fluid to help them work their way into the cervix. If there's a paucity of semen, most of the sperm may flounder and die in the harsh environment of the vagina. Conversely, if there's too much semen, the sperm may exhaust themselves swimming through all of that excess fluid and die in the cervix.

Numerous factors influence how much semen there is in a particular sample. One common reason is sexual intercourse. If a man has sex shortly before giving a semen sample, the volume will be lower than if he had abstained for longer than three days. Also, a low volume of semen—particularly if the sample contains very few sperm—could signal a problem with sperm production or with ejaculation.

After checking the consistency and volume, the technician will examine the semen sample under a microscope. First, he'll scan the sample for any white blood cells, which could signify an infection. Then, he'll turn his attention to the sperm. Because not just any sperm can fertilize an egg, he'll evaluate the sperm for three different characteristics: their overall number, their ability to move, and their shape, or morphology.

Most people realize that a man's semen must contain a sufficient number of motile sperm if fertilization is to occur. As was mentioned before, out of the millions of sperm ejaculated, only a few hundred make it all of the way to the uterus. So it only stands to reason that the greater the number of sperm (up to a certain point), the greater is the chance that at least one of the little travelers will meet and fertilize an egg. Most doctors today feel that a man needs to have at least 20 million motile sperm in each milliliter of ejaculate, and about 60 million motile sperm in the entire sample, if he's to be considered as having normal fertility. This is a good ballpark figure, to be sure. But you'd be wrong to cling to this figure too tightly.

Experts are now realizing that the number of sperm may be much less important than was first thought. Over the years, reports have surfaced that described men who had sperm counts below 10 million and yet who were able to initiate a pregnancy. Furthermore, in the 1970s, some doctors were star-

tled to learn that about 20% of the men requesting vasectomies—and, if they were requesting vasectomies, they most likely had fathered children—had sperm counts that were less than
20 million.[22] This information has triggered the thought that a
couple's fertility is relative: a man's low sperm count may be of
no consequence if his wife is very fertile.

Even more important than the number of sperm is how well
the sperm that are available can move around. After all, if a sperm
is ever going to make it out of the vagina and cervix and into the
fallopian tubes, it has to be able to move. To evaluate this quality
in sperm, the technician will watch to see how many of the sperm
are swimming in a purposeful, progressive manner. Every semen
sample contains at least some sperm that either aren't moving or
that are moving erratically. What's important here is the percentage. In general, to be considered normal, at least 50% of the
sperm in any one sample need to be moving well.

But the evaluation doesn't end here. The technician will
look to see how *well* the sperm are moving, and then he'll assign
the sperm a numerical score, or grade. For example, if the sperm
are simply wiggling in place, he'll assign the sperm a grade 1; if
the sperm are moving forward slowly, or if their route is erratic,
he'll assign a grade 2; if the sperm are moving forward fairly
quickly and maintaining a straight path, he'll assign a grade 3;
and, if the sperm are zipping along at a rapid rate in a straight
line, he'll assign a grade 4. For the most part, the higher the
grade, the greater is the chance that the sperm will be capable of
fertilizing an egg.

The last part of the semen analysis involves an examination
of the shape, or morphology, of the sperm. Again, the morphology of the sperm is more important than the total number of
sperm. Sperm having certain abnormal shapes can't fertilize an
egg. Normally, a sperm has an oval-shaped head and a long tail.
Aberrations include sperm with elongated heads, coiled tails, or
even two heads. Every man produces some abnormally shaped
sperm. The crucial factor is how many. To be considered fertile,
at least 60% of the sperm in a man's semen sample should have a
normal shape.

If you find out that your partner's semen analysis is abnormal or borderline, don't panic. Remember that analysis results can vary, sometimes dramatically, from month to month. Therefore, repeat the analysis once or twice more before you draw any conclusions about your partner's ability to initiate a pregnancy. If a repeat semen analysis shows a deficiency of sperm, the doctor may wish to perform additional studies. For example, blood levels of FSH, LH, prolactin, and testosterone may help pinpoint the cause of the problem. Another useful test involves testing the semen for fructose, a type of sugar normally found in semen. If the semen contains very few or no sperm, and no fructose, then there's a good chance that a blockage in the reproductive system is causing the problem. In a few cases, the doctor may wish to perform a testicular biopsy. By taking a tiny bit of tissue from one testicle, the doctor can gain further information about your partner's production of sperm. For example, he'll learn whether the cells that manufacture sperm are even present. If none of these vital sperm producers exist, there's no hope that the man will ever produce sperm. If these cells are present, and if sperm in various stages of maturation are also present, then the doctor could reasonably conclude that the lack of sperm in the ejaculate was due to a blockage in the transportation system.

Other than a semen analysis, your doctor may recommend that you and your partner undergo additional tests to make sure that your partner's sperm can easily penetrate cervical mucus, and that they can also pierce and fertilize an egg. The two tests used to determine this are the hamster egg penetration test (also called the sperm penetration test and the hamster zona-free egg penetration test) and the cervical mucus–sperm interaction test.

Hamster Egg Penetration Test

In a nutshell, this test analyzes whether a man's sperm can actually penetrate and fertilize an egg. As you may realize, it's not practical to perform this test using a human egg. The only time doctors actually watch fertilization of a human egg is during *in vitro* fertilization. Because this is just a test of fertilization potential, the test is performed on hamster eggs.

I know this sounds strange, and no, people can't actually impregnate hamsters. For fertilization to occur, the egg must divide in a certain way, and that doesn't happen here. Furthermore, the eggs of every species have a protective covering, called a *zona pellucida*, which keeps "foreign" sperm from penetrating. That's why, to see if a human sperm can penetrate a hamster egg, technicians must first remove the outer layer, or zona, from the hamster eggs. They then take 20 to 30 of these zona-free eggs and mix them with a sample of sperm. After letting the mixture incubate for a certain period of time, they check to see how many eggs the sperm penetrated.

Most doctors feel that, to consider a man fertile, the man's sperm should penetrate over 10% of the eggs. If the sperm penetrate fewer than 10% of the eggs, some doctors will conclude that the man's sperm is significantly hindering a couple's chances at conception.

However, there are several problems with that conclusion, and, indeed, with the test in general. Besides the fact that the test costs between $400 and $700, the value of the results is a matter of controversy. For starters, the results can vary depending on how the sperm were handled before being mixed with the eggs, and how long the eggs and sperm remained in contact. There is no set standard for this, and it can vary between labs. And finally, it's debatable as to how pertinent the results of the test are.

To begin with, for conception to occur, a sperm must drill through the tough outer layer, or zona, of the egg. This is perhaps its most difficult task. But, the eggs used in this test are zona-free; therefore, the results don't reflect whether or not the sperm could penetrate the zona of a human egg if it were to confront one. In addition, many doctors question whether the results of this test can provide any more information about male fertility than can a semen analysis. For example, some doctors have found that the hamster test was a poorer predictor of whether or not an egg could be fertilized through *in vitro* fertilization or the GIFT procedure than was a standard semen analysis.[23] What seems to be the best predictor is if the sperm, when analyzed, are moving forward in a straight line.[24]

So, if your doctor wants to perform this test, you should seriously question whether it is necessary. Besides being out as much as $700, you could end up needlessly discouraged about your chances of ever becoming pregnant except through the use of donor sperm. So, think about it, talk with your doctor, and perhaps do further research before deciding whether this test is necessary for you.

Sperm Penetration Tests

Depending upon the results of your postcoital test, the doctor may wish to perform a couple of other tests involving your cervical mucus and your partner's sperm. If the postcoital test showed very few, or no, sperm, one would naturally wonder whether the sperm were dying before they could penetrate the mucus and enter the cervix, or whether something in the mucus was killing them. There are a couple of tests that can help determine this.

The first test is called a sperm-migration test. For this test, a technician would simply drop a small amount of your cervical mucus on a glass slide, cover the mucus with a coverslip, and then apply a small amount of semen along the edge of the coverslip. Three or four hours later, the technician would check the sample under a microscope to see whether any of the sperm had invaded the mucus and, if so, how far they had traveled. Optimally, the sperm would have penetrated the mucus and evenly distributed themselves throughout the sample. This would show that the sperm have the ability to penetrate, and then survive in, your cervical mucus.

A second test evaluates this same thing, but also examines whether the sperm are capable of scaling the female reproductive tract. For this test, a technician would fill a thin, glass tube with a sample of mucus taken from your cervix. He would then place this thin tube inside a test tube containing a sample of your partner's sperm. The sperm should gravitate toward the mucus and, if everything is normal, begin to swim up the tube, just as if they were swimming up the reproductive tract. After an hour, the technician would measure how far the sperm traveled. Ideally, they would have made it about 30 mm up the tube.

To be truly accurate, the technician would run another test at the same time, this time using a sample of cervical mucus taken either from another woman, or, as more commonly occurs, from a cow. The mucus taken from a cow is very similar to a woman's mucus. This second test, which also uses your partner's sperm, would serve as a basis for comparison to the first test. If the tube with your mucus contained only dead or immobile sperm, then antisperm antibodies could very well be the culprit. The next question is, "Who has the antisperm antibodies? You or your partner?" To answer that question, you'd have to look at the results of the test performed on the cow's mucus. If the sperm in that test traveled up the tube without a problem, then the antibodies are most likely in your mucus. On the other hand, if the sperm in the cow cervical mucus performed about the same as they did in your mucus, then it's likely that your partner is producing his own antisperm antibodies.

*   *   *

To summarize, a man is usually considered fertile if he has about 20 million sperm in each milliliter of semen, if more than 50% of the sperm are moving actively after about 6 hours, and if at least 60% of the sperm have a normal shape. Remember, though, that these values are not absolute. Besides the fact that a man's semen analysis can show dramatically different results from month to month, the results themselves are all relative. Even if a man has a fairly poor semen analysis, if the woman is particularly fertile, then that couple may not have a problem conceiving. When age is a factor, though, you need to consider that you may not be as fertile as you once were. Therefore, if you have postponed parenthood, and your partner has a borderline or abnormal semen analysis, you may not want to delay seeking medical help to become pregnant.

The Final Evaluation

The final test of an infertility workup is perhaps the most involved. This test, or procedure, is a laparoscopy. This procedure involves inserting a slender, telescopelike instrument through a tiny incision in your belly button. This instrument, which has a light on one end, allows the doctor to peer into your pelvic cavity and actually see, firsthand, your reproductive organs. By doing so, he can look for endometriosis, which no other test will reveal. He can also search your pelvic cavity for any adhesions or scar tissue that might be binding your fallopian tubes.

The laparoscope allows the doctor to scrutinize every inch of your reproductive organs from the outside; he can even gently lift the ovaries and uterus, peering underneath for any dot of endometriosis. This procedure complements the hysterosalpingogram; the hysterosalpingogram gives a silhouette of the inside of your reproductive organs, while the laparoscopy reveals the status of the outside of these same organs.

The best time to perform the laparoscopy is debatable. Some doctors like to perform the laparoscopy in the first half of the menstrual cycle, to avoid disrupting a pregnancy. Other doctors like to perform the procedure after ovulation has occurred. This way, they can look for a corpus luteum, which would help prove that ovulation did, indeed, occur.

To have a laparoscopy performed, you'd have to go to a hospital; however, you'd most likely be admitted as an outpatient, meaning that you'd be able to go home within a few hours of the procedure. Most people undergoing this procedure receive a general anesthetic. Once you're appropriately anesthetized, the doctor would make a tiny incision in your belly button through which he'd instill carbon dioxide gas. This gas serves to inflate the abdomen, enlarging the doctor's work space and allowing for better visualization of the reproductive organs. To increase visualization even more, the operating room table will be tilted head down. This slanting position causes the intestines to slide away from the reproductive organs, opening up the pelvic cavity for an even better view.

The doctor would then insert the laparoscope through the incision in your belly button and begin his visual search of your peritoneal cavity. If he spotted any sign of endometriosis or scar tissue, he could use a laser or an electric probe to vaporize the harmful tissue. If necessary, he could even attach surgical instruments to the end of the laparoscope and cut away adhesions and scar tissue.

While your doctor has your fallopian tubes in site, he'll most likely inject a dye solution through your uterine cavity and watch as it flows out the ends of the fallopian tubes. This way, he'll know for certain that the fallopian tubes are open. If the tubes show an obstruction, the doctor will be able to examine them immediately.

After completing all of the necessary tasks, the doctor would then stitch the incision closed. The incision is very tiny, small enough, in fact, to be covered by a Band-Aid. It should cause very little pain and, once healed, will probably be invisible.

Laparoscopy is fairly safe, and you should recover quickly. However, just as with any other procedure, there are possible complications. These include complications related to the anesthesia as well as pelvic infection, bleeding, and damage to the intestines or bladder. Including both the doctor's and hospital's fees, the procedure costs between $3000 and $5000.

Hysteroscopy

While you're under anesthesia for the laparoscopy, the doctor may want to examine the inside of your uterus. This procedure, called a hysteroscopy, involves inserting a second instrument through your vagina and cervix and into your uterus. This instrument, called a hysteroscope, allows the doctor to examine directly the inside of the uterus for anything that could interfere with pregnancy, such as fibroids, polyps, or scar tissue. (Remember that the laparoscope only allows for visualization of the outside of the reproductive organs.) This procedure would be especially important if the hysterosalpingogram hinted at any type of uterine abnormality. Also, if you've ever had an IUD, or if you've ever undergone an abortion or D & C, you're at greater risk for having scar tissue inside your uterus, so it could be important that you have a hysteroscopy performed.

Again, complications are rare, but they can include pain, a lacerated cervix, a perforated uterus, infection, endometriosis, and complications from the anesthesia.

*   *   *

There you have it, the complete basic infertility workup. It seems extensive, but, if performed in an orderly, methodical manner, you can put all of this behind you within a couple of months. For example, in one month, you could have the postcoital test performed during the first half of your cycle. Then, during the second half of the same cycle, you could have the ultrasound performed, followed by the endometrial biopsy and hormone levels. Your partner could also have a semen analysis performed some time that same month. Then, the next month, you could complete the workup with the hysterosalpingogram, laparoscopy, and hysteroscopy. If all of the tests were performed correctly, you'd have more than a 90% chance of knowing what, if anything, was causing you to have a delay in conception. Knowing that, you could proceed with any necessary treatment, and hopefully be that much closer to pregnancy.

9

Improving the Odds

At this point, you may not even know when you want to conceive, much less whether or not you'll have a problem and require treatment. But, by postponing pregnancy, you're increasing your risk for infertility. Therefore, if you wish to make a truly informed decision about whether, or how long, to delay your plans for parenthood, you need to consider the treatment options that will be available if you eventually have a problem conceiving. Simply learning about your risks for infertility, without learning what can be done to treat a problem, is like buying a house in an area with unstable soil without knowing what you can do if the house develops a foundation problem.

To further illustrate, there has been much excited talk about the new technological treatments that have allowed women who, in years past, would never have been able to have children to conceive and carry a child to term. But, instead of simply relying on these seemingly miraculous treatments as insurance for when your biological clock's batteries begin to run low, you need to know—in advance—what these procedures really are. How much do they cost? What are the chances for success? What, exactly, do these procedures entail? In other words, will these procedures really be an option for you?

Treatments for the Infertile

You may already know, or at least suspect, that you have a problem that may interfere with your becoming pregnant. For example, you may have erratic periods and suspect that you're not ovulating normally. Or, your partner may have had a severe case of mumps during adolescence, and you suspect that his sperm count may be less than optimal. Even if you don't have any clue as to whether or not you have a problem, an infertility workup could turn up an abnormality. If that occurs, what can be done?

Following is a brief discussion of some treatments used to correct the most common fertility disorders. While reading this, keep in mind that, if you've postponed trying to become pregnant, you won't have a lot of time to waste, especially if you want to have more than one child. While many of these conventional treatments are effective, most take time—time that you may not have. That's why, if you eventually learn that you're having difficulty becoming pregnant, you'll want to move quickly to more aggressive treatments, which we'll discuss in more detail later in the chapter.

Ovulatory Dysfunction

Let's say that, after having an infertility evaluation, you discover that you're not ovulating correctly. What can be done? Actually, lots of things, but exactly what will depend upon *why* you're not ovulating. If it's because your thyroid hormone is out of whack, then treatment will focus on bringing that hormone into line. If the doctor discovers that you have an elevated level of the hormone prolactin, then he will no doubt prescribe a medication called bromocriptine, or Parlodel. This drug is very effective in decreasing the production of prolactin, after which ovulation will most likely resume. Most of the time, though, lack of ovulation is due to some subtle imbalance between the hormones directly responsible for ovulation. For example, if your body isn't producing enough FSH in the first half of the menstrual cycle, the eggs won't mature, and you won't ovulate. That's where some of the well-known "fertility drugs" come in.

Probably the most well-known, and widely prescribed, drug used to treat infertility is clomiphene citrate, which goes by the trade name Clomid or Serophene. Clomiphene acts on the pituitary gland to increase the production of FSH. This extra FSH sees to it that one or more eggs mature in preparation of ovulation. Not only is this helpful if you don't ovulate at all, it also helps regulate ovulation. For example, let's say you ovulate late, like day 18 or 19 of your cycle. Taking clomiphene will most likely cause you to ovulate on day 14, instead. Clomiphene can also be a remedy for a shortened luteal phase. By stimulating FSH production, the drug helps ensure proper development of the follicle; and a mature, healthy follicle is more likely to secrete the hormones necessary for maintaining the endometrial lining.

Clomiphene is taken orally on days five through nine (or days three through seven) of a menstrual cycle. Most doctors start out by prescribing one tablet (50 mg) a day, but the dosage may climb to as many as four tablets, or 200 mg, a day, depending upon whether or not ovulation is occurring. A benefit of clomiphene is that it is fairly mild, meaning that women who take it don't require as close monitoring as do women taking more potent ovulation stimulating agents. It's also fairly inexpensive, at least as far as fertility medications go. Clomiphene costs about $5 to $6 per tablet; so if you're taking one 50-mg tablet daily for five days each cycle, your monthly cost would be $25 to $30.

The fertility enhancing effects of clomiphene can only be maintained for six to eight cycles. After that, some of clomiphene's other actions begin to dominate, which can actually hinder fertility. For example, while clomiphene encourages the pituitary gland to secrete more FSH, it also interferes with the efforts of estrogen. As you already know, estrogen prompts the cervix to produce the mucus that's so hospitable to sperm. Without enough estrogen, the cervix tends to produce mucus that is thick, sticky, in short supply, and difficult for sperm to penetrate. Besides that, clomiphene may also interfere with estrogen's actions on the endometrium. As you may recall, estrogen is partially responsible for making sure that the endometrial lining develops appropriately. If clomiphene interferes with estrogen's actions here, a luteal phase defect could result. (Yes, you're reading correctly. Just a minute ago, I said that clomiphene is sometimes used to *treat* a luteal phase defect. It's paradoxical: at times, it's used to treat a luteal phase defect; at other times, it causes a defect.)

The obvious solution to these problems is to give the woman a supplement of estrogen after she's stopped taking clomiphene and before she's ovulated. But it really isn't that simple. Although the extra estrogen may help improve the quality of the cervical mucus and encourage endometrial development, it can also disrupt the timing of ovulation, which wouldn't be in your best interest if you were trying to conceive.

Something else to consider is that although 80% of the women with ovulatory disorders who take clomiphene begin to ovulate, only about 40% of those ultimately conceive.[1] The success rate is higher, though, if lack of ovulation is the only problem. But, if you've postponed childbearing, age is one more factor with which you'll have to contend.

Many doctors—particularly those untrained in the area of reproductive endocrinology—think of clomiphene as a cure-all for infertility and prescribe it to almost any woman who has difficulty conceiving. But clomiphene isn't a cure-all. If you ovulate normally, clomiphene is *not* the drug for you. Not only will it not facilitate pregnancy, its side effects could very well interfere with your efforts to conceive. Even if you've a proven defect in the ovulatory process, if you've put off trying to conceive until your mid to late 30s you won't want to spend too much time taking clomiphene. Rather, it could be a good idea to move on to something stronger. And that something stronger is human menopausal gonadotropin, which is known by the trade names Pergonal or Metrodin.

Pergonal contains a small amount of LH, but it's primarily FSH itself—the hormone that the body naturally produces to stimulate the development of follicles inside the ovaries. It's not a synthetic preparation; it's the pure hormone that has been obtained from the urine of postmenopausal women. (After menopause, women secrete large amounts of FSH and LH in their urine.) When the hormone is injected, it rushes to the ovaries, causing them to snap to attention and begin working overtime developing eggs for ovulation. That's what makes Pergonal so powerful. Instead of acting on the pituitary gland to affect hormone levels indirectly, as clomiphene does, it acts directly on the organs in question: the ovaries.

As you already know, though, FSH doesn't control the process of ovulation single-handedly. For the ovaries to release their grip on the ripe eggs, they need a jolt of LH. So, after a woman takes Pergonal for a certain number of days, she receives an injection of a medication called human chorionic gonadotropin, or HCG. The sudden infusion of HCG acts like the normal mid-cycle surge of LH, causing the ripe eggs to break free from the ovary. In most instances, not just one but several eggs leave the ovary for a trip down the fallopian tube.

To keep this burst of HCG pure and undiluted by any LH the woman's body might produce, some doctors recommend that the woman take injections of another medication, known by the trade name Lupron, either before or while she's taking Pergonal. Lupron blocks the body's production of LH, and ensures that any naturally produced LH won't disrupt egg development or cause ovulation to occur before the eggs are completely mature. This way, everything is controlled; the eggs won't be pushed out of the ovary until they're prime candidates for fertilization.

This all sounds great, doesn't it? Here's a medication that will force your ovaries to release several eggs at once, and, to further increase your chances for conception, you'll know exactly when you'll ovulate. But such monumental actions don't come easily. Although Pergonal is one of the major therapies used by many infertility clinics, you need to consider exactly what's involved.

To begin with, all of the medications we just discussed must be given by injection on a daily basis. That means you'll have to make sure that your partner, or someone else, is available on those key days to give you your shot. If either you or your partner travel as a part of your jobs, this could turn into a major hassle. Furthermore, for several days in the middle of your cycle, you'll have to go to your doctor's office each day for a blood test to check your estrogen level and an ultrasound to monitor the development of ovarian follicles. There's no way to get around this. Pergonal is strong medicine, and the doctor must keep close tabs on your ovaries to make sure they don't balloon out of control with this sudden infusion of hormone. With proper monitoring, though, this rampant stimulation, known as hyperstimulation, rarely occurs.

To give you some idea of what your life would be like if you were to take Pergonal, here's a breakdown of a typical cycle. Before beginning anything, you'd visit your doctor's office for an ultrasound to make sure your ovaries were free and clear of unruptured follicles. If it's determined that your ovaries are starting with a clean slate, you'd begin taking Pergonal on day three of your cycle (which is three days after the beginning of your last menstrual period). For the next three days, you'd receive an injection of Pergonal, probably two or three ampules at a time. Then, on the fourth to sixth day, you'd go to your doctor's office for another ultrasound and a blood test for estrogen.

The ultrasound will reveal the number of follicles developing on your ovaries as well as the size of the follicles. The blood level of estrogen will help to back up that information. A follicle that's ready to release a mature egg produces about 200 pg/ml of estrogen; therefore, by comparing your blood level of estrogen with the number of follicles visible on ultrasound, the doctor will gain some idea as to when the eggs are ready for ovulation. In addition, the results of these tests reveal how your ovaries are responding to the Pergonal. If your ovaries are barely eking out a follicle or two, the doctor will no doubt increase your dosage.

Therefore, the afternoon after the blood test and the ultrasound, you'd check with the doctor's office to see how much Pergonal to take in your next dose. You'd keep up this routine of injecting Pergonal (and Lupron, too, if your doctor prescribed it) every day, and visiting the doctor's office every day, until one or two of the follicles reached prime size (about 16 mm or more) and your serum estrogen level climbed, on average, to between 450 and 900 pg/ml. Typically, this would take about nine or ten days from the beginning of your cycle.

If it happened that your estrogen level climbed to greater than 2000 pg/ml, you'd probably have to stop everything and let your ovaries return to normal without ever ovulating. Triggering ovulation in such hyperstimulated ovaries could have dire consequences for your ovaries as well as your general health. But, in most instances, this won't happen if you're being monitored every day as you go along. So, when everything is right and your ovaries are at their peak, you'd stop taking Pergonal and receive an injection of HCG. About 36 hours after receiving this jolt of hormone, your ovaries would release the mature eggs, thus causing ovulation.

Of course, developing and releasing eggs is just half of the process. Now the eggs have to get fertilized. Knowing when you'll ovulate will help you pin down the best time for intercourse, which is, in general, the day you receive HCG and then every day until an ultrasound shows that at least one follicle has ruptured and released an egg. Some doctors feel that they can further increase the chances for fertilization by performing intrauterine insemination using the partner's sperm. Their reasoning, first of all, is that intrauterine insemination prepares the semen so that only the most viable sperm are used. Next, intrauterine insemination bypasses the cervix, thus relieving the sperm of the chore of penetrating the cervical mucus, and places them high in the uterus close to the fallopian tubes. Of course, the downside is that, by bypassing the cervix, the sperm may only survive a matter of hours, instead of a matter of days. Therefore, the best time to perform intrauterine insemination is after ovulation has occurred, which would be revealed by the image of an empty follicle on ultrasound. To improve the odds even further, some doctors choose to perform two inseminations: one just before ovulation is expected to occur, and another just after.

Once you've ovulated, you're still not free to take the rest of the month off. Because some women who take Pergonal don't produce enough progesterone to maintain the endometrium, your doctor may want you to take progesterone supplements—in the form of daily injections or vaginal suppositories—beginning a few days after ovulation. This progesterone boost will see to it that your endometrium is ready and willing to receive a fertilized egg if one should arrive.

Finally, about 2 weeks after ovulation, you'd receive a pregnancy test that would tell you whether or not your efforts to achieve a pregnancy were successful. At that time, if a pregnancy test is positive, you'd continue taking progesterone for 6 more weeks, by which time the placenta should be developed enough to produce all the progesterone your body needs. If the pregnancy test is negative, you'd first repeat the test, and then, if it was still negative, you'd simply stop the progesterone and wait for your period. You'd then most likely take the next month off from Pergonal treatment to allow your ovaries—not to mention your injection-sore hips and your strained emotions—a chance to recover before starting the routine again.

All of this therapy doesn't come cheap. A single ampule of Pergonal costs from $40 to $50; depending upon how many amps of Pergonal you take a day, your monthly bill for medication alone could run from $800 to $1500. The daily ultrasounds and estrogen levels will add another $800 to $1000 to the cost, bringing the monthly total to $1600 to $2500. And that doesn't include the doctor's charge or the costs of Lupron or progesterone, if used.

Now that you're aware of the cost and intensiveness of Pergonal therapy, you need to realize that Pergonal isn't a cure-all. The success rate of the therapy depends on what it's treating. When used to treat women who don't ovulate or menstruate because of some abnormality in hormone production, the success rate is quite high. For example, in one study of 279 such patients, 82% conceived after having received Pergonal. But, when evaluated in relation to the patients' age, the success rates aren't quite so high. While women younger than age 35 had more than a 95% chance of conceiving during six treatment cycles, women older than age 35 had only a 60% chance.[2] Still, those are better results than the same group of women could have expected if they'd been taking clomiphene. In a study of women with the same disorder who took clomiphene, the women younger than age 35 had a 55% chance for conceiving, while women older than age 35 had a very poor chance for becoming pregnant at all.[3]

Although Pergonal is often used to treat women with unexplained infertility, it has not been shown to be particularly effective. Nor has it been particularly effective in inducing pregnancy in women who only have a luteal phase defect or poor mucus production to explain their difficulties conceiving. In fact, when Pergonal is used to treat women with such disorders, the pregnancy rate is a measly 12%.[4] This may be better than nothing, though, considering that a control group in this study had an even lower pregnancy rate. At the same time, though, you need to be aware that another study found that women who had unexplained infertility and who received no treatment had a 14% pregnancy rate. This is 2% *higher* than the pregnancy rate of the group taking Pergonal.[5] To make matters worse, women who conceive on Pergonal—regardless of their diagnosis beforehand—still have to face a 21.5% miscarriage rate, the same miscarriage rate faced by the general population.[6]

And finally, if you ever do decide to pursue Pergonal therapy, you need to be aware that its beneficial effects are time-limited. Most pregnancies following ovulation induction with

Pergonal occur within the first three cycles. In fact, the greatest chance for pregnancy with Pergonal occurs after just the first cycle.

Although this information might be depressing enough, you also need to consider the possible side effects of Pergonal. As was already mentioned, it's possible for your ovaries to balloon out of control under the effects of Pergonal; however, this risk is slight as long as you're monitored carefully. There's also a chance, because of Pergonal's ability to cause the release of more than one egg, that you'd have a multiple birth. However, 80% of the women who deliver a baby after taking Pergonal deliver a single baby. Even in women who have multiple births, 75% of the time it's only twins.

And finally, what about long-term risks? Unfortunately, the jury's still out on whether or not there are any long-term risks. At present, women who have taken Pergonal don't seem to be at any greater risk for developing breast or endometrial cancer than do other women. However, it's still too soon to say for sure. Many carcinogens, such as radiation or other toxic substances, require years before their effects become noticeable. Therefore, it will be another 10 to 15 years before experts learn whether Pergonal causes any long-term damage. For now, though, it seems to be safe.

It also seems to be safe for the babies conceived through the aid of Pergonal. These infants seem to be normal and healthy, and they have no greater risk for birth defects than do other infants. Their pattern of growth and development also appears normal.[7]

In summary, Pergonal therapy is extremely intensive, not to mention expensive. But, for women who have ovulatory dysfunction, it can make the difference between becoming pregnant and remaining childless. If you simply have unexplained infertility, or if aging seems to have taken its toll on your ability to reproduce, its effectiveness is debatable. Some doctors swear by it, but the decision is ultimately yours. Now that you have the facts and figures, if you're ever faced with receiving such treatment, you'll have something on which to base your decision.

Tubal Disorders

After having an infertility workup, you might discover that your fallopian tubes aren't functioning as they should. It could be that scar tissue in your peritoneum is anchoring your tubes in place so they can't pick up an ovulating egg. It's also possible that a previous infection inflamed the interior of your tubes, causing the sides of the tubes to stick together and create a blockage. The most common site for an infection to take root, though, is at the ends of the tubes near the ovaries. This is unfortunate, because a problem here affects the delicate, flowerlike filaments that fringe the ends of the tubes; the inflammation and resultant scarring cause the filaments to clump together. When this happens, the filaments can't spread wide and sweep an egg into the fallopian tube. Also, when severe, the scarring can completely seal off the ends of the tubes. Not only does this preclude an egg from ever entering the tube, it also prevents normal fallopian tube secretions from draining out the ends of the tubes. As a result, the secretions pool inside the fallopian tubes, causing the tubes to swell; this condition is known as hydrosalpinx. Still another disorder that can afflict your fallopian tubes is endometriosis. The causes and treatment of endometriosis were discussed in detail in Chapter 5.

Whether treatment can resolve these problems depends on a variety of factors. First and foremost, it depends on the severity of damage. Remember that the fallopian tubes are more than just conduits: they are active participants in the process of fertilization. For example, the insides of the fallopian tubes contain cells that secrete fluids for nourishing an egg on its journey to the uterus. If a past infection destroyed those cells, then the prognosis for resolving the resultant infertility is worse than if peritoneal scar tissue is simply binding the tubes.

Another factor that affects the prognosis is the site of the damage; occlusion at the ends of the tubes has a poorer prognosis than does damage to the center of the tube. In addition, the more of the tube that's been damaged, the slimmer are the chances for recovery. And, finally, the prognosis depends upon the skill of the surgeon trying to correct the damage. Realize that the fallopian tubes are exquisitely small and extremely delicate. For this reason, if you ever need to have surgery on your fallopian tubes, you need to take pains to make sure that your surgeon is specialized in microsurgery and that he knows how to remove adhesions without causing further scarring. The methods used to remove the scar tissue vary with the circumstances, but surgeons often use a laser to vaporize adhesions and scar tissue.

If the fallopian tube is still intact and functional, and the only problem is scar tissue that is anchoring the tube and preventing it from catching an ovulating egg, then the outlook is good. A skilled surgeon should be able to release the tube from the adhesions, which would allow the reproductive process to become more normal. As long as the tubes themselves aren't damaged, women with this type of problem have about a 60% chance of conceiving after surgery.

Also, if the tubes are blocked near the uterus, a new procedure, called transcervical balloon tuboplasty, has proved promising. The procedure, which costs about $3000, involves sliding a catheter through your cervix up to the point of the blockage. The doctor then inflates a tiny balloon in the catheter's tip, which pushes the blocking tissue out of the way. One medical study showed that 71 of 77 women undergoing this tuboplasty procedure had at least one tube opened as a result. Of those, 22 later became pregnant.[8] Doctors estimate that the tube should remain open for about 18 months following the tuboplasty.

However, if scar tissue has completely blocked the ends of the fallopian tubes near the ovaries, things may not be so easily resolved. This portion of the fallopian tube is extremely delicate, and surgery could further damage the fragile filaments. Besides that, severely damaged filaments typically indicate that the interior of the tubes is severely damaged as well. If so, the chances are poor that surgery will allow the tubes to recover to the extent necessary for pregnancy to occur. Again, the chances for success are directly related to the severity of damage.

For example, a study of 130 women whose fallopian tubes were scarred at the ends revealed that 30% were able to conceive and carry a baby to term after having corrective surgery.[9] But, in another study of 142 women whose scarring was severe enough to cause hydrosalpinx, only 19% were able to conceive and carry to term.[10] You also need to realize that, after any kind of tubal surgery, you'll have an increased risk for having an ectopic pregnancy.

Even if your tubes are extensively damaged, there's still hope for pregnancy. As long as your uterus is intact, and your ovaries are healthy, you could still become pregnant through *in vitro* fertilization. This procedure is discussed in detail later in this chapter.

Cervical and Uterine Disorders

The cervix and uterus rarely cause infertility, but "rarely" doesn't mean "never." If one of these organs turns out to be hindering your attempts at pregnancy, you'll want to know what can be done.

As you already know, the main problems with the cervix involve either hostile cervical mucus, such as from an infection or antisperm antibodies, or a deformed shape. (For a detailed discussion of the treatment of antisperm antibodies, refer to Chapter 8.) For many cervical problems, the treatment of choice is to bypass the cervix and instill sperm directly into the uterus. This is known as intrauterine insemination.

Intrauterine insemination is a fairly simple procedure where the doctor places a washed sample of your partner's sperm high in your uterus. This bypasses any roadblocks the cervix might erect, and positions the sperm so that they're well on their way to the fallopian tubes. Please note, though, that the doctor places *sperm* in the uterus, not semen. In actuality, semen isn't the greatest environment for sperm to reside in for more than a few hours. In addition, injecting semen directly into the uterine cavity would cause terrific uterine cramps. During normal intercourse, the sperm shake off the semen in the cervix. But, since intrauterine insemination bypasses this stage, the sperm are removed from the semen in a laboratory procedure known as "washing."

Sperm washing serves a couple of purposes. By removing the semen, the sperm become more active and mobile and can live longer. Also, the washing prepares the sperm for the process of fertilizing an egg. Believe it or not, sperm don't exit from the male ready and willing to fertilize an egg. A little prep work must be done first: specifically, a sperm must discard a caplike covering from its head. This prep work—known as capacitation—normally occurs in the female genital tract. Because intrauterine insemination bypasses much of this territory, capacitation must take place in the laboratory.

Once the sperm are washed clean of semen, they are immersed in another liquid. When everything is ready, the doctor would draw up the sperm solution into a catheter. With you lying on an examination table with your feet in stirrups, the doctor would insert the catheter through your vagina and cervix and up into your uterus. He would then inject the solution, introducing your partner's sperm into your uterine cavity. Within minutes, the sperm could be in the fallopian tubes.

Because intrauterine insemination allows the sperm to flood the fallopian tubes within minutes, and because the sperm no longer have the luxury of lounging in the cervix for a couple of days, it's best to undergo this procedure shortly after ovulation has occurred. If an egg is waiting in the fallopian tube, intrauterine insemination has a much greater chance for being successful.

A single insemination costs approximately $100 to $150. Because the odds of becoming pregnant during any one cycle of artificial insemination are less than they are for normal inter-course, it could take several months—and several insemina-tions—before you conceive.

Another possible problem with the cervix is one that, al-though it wouldn't interfere with pregnancy, could prevent your carrying a child to term. This problem, which is known as an incompetent cervix, occurs when the cervix is too weak to sup-port the weight of a developing fetus. As the weight of the fetus increases, the cervix stretches thinner until it finally dilates, causing a miscarriage. A typical remedy for an incompetent cer-vix involves placing a running suture, called a purse-string su-ture, along the edge of the cervix once you become pregnant. The suture is pulled tight, which gives the cervix more support. When the time for delivery approaches, the suture is removed and the delivery occurs naturally.

When the uterus is a problem, it's often because of some malformation. Whether or not this will cause infertility depends upon the degree of the deformity. If the deformity is slight, then fertility may not be affected at all. But if the deformity is severe, and the uterine cavity is extremely small, then it could very well put an end to your plans for pregnancy. Occasionally, depend-ing upon the type and degree of deformity, surgery might be able to correct the problem. For example, when the uterus is divided into two cavities by a thin wall of tissue, surgery can usually remove this tissue and create an excellent chance for pregnancy. On the average, though, uterine problems are very difficult, if not impossible, to resolve.

The uterus might also be a problem if it contains scar tissue, such as that resulting from a past infection or a D & C. In many instances, surgery can remove the scar tissue and restore fertil-ity. Fibroid tumors or polyps may also interfere with pregnancy, although this rarely occurs. If these unwanted growths are a culprit in foiled fertility, surgery can remove them. But, resort to surgery only after your doctor has ruled out all other causes for a fertility problem, and only if he's sure that the growths are inter-fering with your attempts at pregnancy.

Male Infertility

Last but not least, you need to consider that your partner might cause or contribute to your having difficulty conceiving. For 25% to 50% of all infertile couples, the male is at least part of the problem.[11] As you already know, to be considered normally fertile, a man must have a certain number of normally shaped sperm that are moving quickly in a straight line. A problem with the number, shape, or motility of the sperm could be enough to hinder fertility.

Unfortunately, treating the problem of male infertility is more than a little tricky. Occasionally, a doctor might discover a straightforward cause for infertility that can be treated through medication or surgery. Such causes include a genitourinary infection, an underactive thyroid gland, an endocrine disorder, or an anatomical defect, such as a urethra that exits on the underside of the penis. Another treatable cause of infertility is a blockage in the sperm transportation system. Such a blockage— whether due to a past infection or a congenital defect—would keep the sperm locked inside the epididymis, preventing them from exiting the body. In this instance, microsurgery can often clear the blockage and restore fertility.

Most of the time, though, the reason behind a man's infertility is unknown. Most infertile men appear healthy and, other than an abnormal semen analysis, have absolutely no symptoms. That's what makes treating male infertility so difficult: if you don't know what's wrong, you can't fix it.

One possible cause of male infertility that has received a lot of attention is the varicocele. A varicocele is, essentially, a varicose vein of the testicle. Somewhere between 20% and 40% of all infertile men have varicoceles. Knowing this, some experts have suggested that varicoceles somehow cause, or at least contribute to, a man's infertility. Exactly how this may occur isn't certain. Some have theorized that the varicocele causes blood to pool in the testicle, which, in turn, causes the temperature in the testicle to rise to a level that inhibits sperm production. Regardless, many experts have claimed that removing the varicocele can stimulate sperm production.

This could be exciting news, especially in light of the fact that doctors are often helpless to do *anything* about male infertility. But, there's another side to the story. Although 20% to 40% of all infertile men have varicoceles, so do about 20% of the men who have normal fertility. For this reason alone, one can't say that a varicocele in itself causes infertility. But there's more.

A study published in the *British Medical Journal* examined 651 infertile couples in which the man had a varicocele. Slightly fewer than half of the men—283 to be exact—had the varicocele surgically removed. The remaining 368 men did not. At the end of a year's time, 30% of the couples had conceived, regardless of whether or not the man had had the varicocele removed. At the end of the second year, 45% of all of the couples had conceived. Again, whether or not the man had had the varicocele surgically removed didn't influence whether or not the couple became pregnant.[12]

And besides the fact that the results are less than convincing, the surgery used to remove the varicocele is expensive; the procedure costs from $1300 to $4000. For these reasons, you and your partner may wish to think long and hard before having this procedure performed.

If your partner's only problem is that he doesn't produce a large quantity of sperm, then there may not be a reason to despair. Remember that how well the sperm are moving is more important than the total number of sperm. In fact, some experts feel that as long as a man's sperm count is above 10 million, then a couple shouldn't have any great difficulty conceiving.[13] Supporting this theory is a study of 386 men who were known to be fertile; 20% of these men had sperm counts below 20 million.[14]

If your partner has a sperm count of 20 million, it would take *longer* for you to conceive than if he had a sperm count of 60 million, but you should be able to conceive *eventually*. However, if you've postponed childbearing, your fertility level may be suboptimal, which would compound the problem. But, because there's no real treatment to augment male fertility, the best initial course of action may be to improve your level of fertility as much as possible. By doing so, your body may be in more of a position to take advantage of the few sperm that are available. Of course, with age working against you, you wouldn't want to devote more than just a few months to this strategy.

Another strategy sometimes used to augment the fertility of a couple that *doesn't* seem to work is intrauterine insemination. Some doctors have felt that by helping the sperm bypass the harsh environment of the vagina and the challenging mucus of the cervix, they can increase the number of sperm that ultimately reach the fallopian tubes. While this would seem to increase the chances for conception, this hasn't really occurred. One reason for this seems to be that when a man's semen contains a decreased number of sperm, or when the sperm are sluggish or abnormally shaped, the sperm tend to have other, unseen abnormalities—abnormalities that may keep them from fertilizing an egg. Knowing this, you can see that simply placing these sperm in the uterus may not be enough for conception to occur.[15]

If your partner's infertility seems to be significantly hindering you chances for conception, most doctors will recommend that you consider receiving artificial insemination with donor sperm.

Artificial Insemination with Donor Sperm

At first, you may have difficulty viewing this as a viable option. After all, you may reason, you wanted to have a baby with your partner, not simply get pregnant by the sperm of someone you don't even know. But this is the wrong attitude to have. Having a baby through the help of donor sperm is really no different from adoption. In fact, it's better in many ways. First, the baby would have half your biologic complement. What's more, by carrying and delivering the baby yourself, you and your partner would have the opportunity to bond with the baby right from the beginning.

Artificial insemination with donor sperm, or DI, is a very real alternative for many couples. In the United States alone, between 6000 and 10,000 babies are born each year as a result of DI.[16] Of course, before choosing this option, you and your partner would have some soul-searching to do. Would both of you be able to accept and love a child who was created with the help of donor sperm? Would you both be able to consider your partner the child's real father? Legally speaking, most states have laws that state implicitly that the *real* father of a child is the man the child lives with, not the man who produced the sperm.

If you choose to go this route, you can rest assured that the insemination is kept completely confidential. Not only would you not be able to learn the identity of the donor, the donor wouldn't be able to learn your identity, either. To further ensure that there are no slipups, some clinics performing DI destroy all records pertaining to the insemination within one year. Since you would already know everything there is to know about the donor's medical history, there's really no reason not to destroy the records. Regardless, though, to reassure yourself that there was no possibility that someone would some day show up and try to make a claim on your child, you'd want to ask the clinic what measures it takes to ensure confidentiality.

Because clinics require donors to have above-average fertility, most donors are young. Also, because many interns and medical students donate sperm—simply because doing so is convenient for them because they work in a medical environment, and also because they are paid a small fee—most donors are of above-average intelligence. And, perhaps most important, the donors must be healthy. All donors receive a thorough medical evaluation to screen for hereditary disease, mental illness, and physical disease. The donors also receive tests to detect the presence of sexually transmitted diseases, including the AIDS virus. Because it can take up to six months after exposure

to the AIDS virus before an AIDS test returns positive, all donated sperm is frozen and stored for six months. After that time,
the donor returns for another AIDS test. Only if that test is still
negative can the sperm be used for insemination.

It's unfortunate that such measures are necessary because
sperm are damaged in the freezing process. The sperm in a
sample that has been frozen and then thawed may have only
half the motility that it had when it was fresh. Naturally, this can
delay the time to conception. To illustrate, one study showed
that the average time to conception for women who ovulated
normally and who were inseminated with fresh semen was 2.8
months. But, for women who were inseminated with frozen
semen, the average time to conception was 5.5 months. To make
matters worse, if the woman required treatment for an ovulatory disorder at the same time she was being inseminated, the
time to conception was even longer. Under these circumstances,
when the women received fresh semen, it took an average of 6.6
months to conceive; when frozen semen was used, it took a
lengthy 22 months before conception occurred.[17] But, the point
is hardly worth arguing. Unless you know the donor, it's imper-
ative that you respect the 6-month lag time between donation
and insemination so that you can avoid any possibility of exposure to the AIDS virus.

If you and your partner decide to undergo DI, the first step
is selecting the donor. Many clinics take care of this for you.
They try their best to match the physical characteristics of the
donor—such as race, hair and eye color, and height—to the
physical characteristics of your partner. The object, of course, is
to select a donor who looks as much like your partner as possible.

Once the donor is selected, the insemination process is relatively simple. After undergoing a minimal workup to make sure
you're ovulating and that your fallopian tubes are open, you'd
maintain a basal body temperature chart or use an ovulation
predictor kit to predict, as accurately as possible, when you'd
ovulate. Once that day is imminent, you'd report to your doc-

tor's office. You'd lie on an examining table with your feet in the stirrups, and the doctor would draw the donor sperm sample into a syringe. He'd then insert the syringe into your vagina, after which he'd squirt the sperm into your cervical area. You'd remain lying flat for about ten minutes to give the sperm a chance to settle in. The doctor may also place a special cap over your cervix to prevent any of the sperm from leaking back into your vagina. After about three hours, you'd be free to remove the cap.

How many DI procedures you'd have to undergo before becoming pregnant varies, depending upon several factors. First of all, women over age 35 who receive DI take significantly longer to conceive than do younger women. And, if your fertility was being hampered by an ovulatory disorder as well, it would take even longer. Finally, women over age 35 who conceive with DI have a significantly greater risk for having a miscarriage once they do conceive.[18] As an example, in one study of 330 couples, 84% of the women younger than age 30 conceived within 12 cycles of donor insemination, whereas only 57% of the women older than age 35 conceived after the same amount of treatment. Also, only 8% of the women between the ages of 26 and 30 had a miscarriage after becoming pregnant with DI, compared to 30% of the women older than age 36.[19]

Going through artificial insemination with donor sperm is understandably stressful. You should be prepared for this going in, realizing that all women feel some degree of stress when undergoing DI. In fact, 25% of the women undergoing DI stop ovulating and develop a luteal phase defect early in the course of treatment.[20] This is almost entirely due to stress. In most instances, everything gets back to normal after just a few months.

*   *   *

All of the treatments discussed have helped many, many women become pregnant. And there's a good chance that, if you ultimately have a problem conceiving, one of these treatments will help solve your infertility problem. But remember, if you've delayed childbearing, time is at a premium. Carefully evaluate the chances of success of any treatment before committing more than just a few months to the regimen. When age is a factor, it's often best not to waste time and to move on to one of the newer technological treatments for infertility.

High-Tech Pregnancy

Strides are being made every day in this area of assisted reproductive technology, allowing many women who thought they'd never have a baby finally conceive. New procedures for promoting pregnancy have come into being. Many have touted these treatments as miracle cures, and, perhaps, they are. But they're also intensive medical procedures.

At this point in your life, it would be easy to sit back and comfort yourself with the fact that sophisticated procedures exist that can help you conceive if you ever have a problem. But then you wouldn't be taking active control over your reproductive health. To make a truly informed decision about childbearing, you need to consider all of your choices. For this reason, you need to have at least a working understanding of what these new, high-tech procedures are all about.

In Vitro Fertilization

In vitro fertilization, or IVF, received national attention in the late 1970s when it was announced that a healthy baby girl had been born as a result of this "test tube" procedure. Since then, thousands of other babies have come into the world because of this seemingly miraculous technology. What is IVF, really? Are babies actually grown in laboratories in test tubes?

No, not exactly. Very simply, to perform an IVF procedure, a doctor retrieves several ripe eggs from a woman's ovaries, places those eggs in a culture dish along with sperm from either her partner or a donor, and then places the mixture in an incubator for a couple of days to allow the eggs to fertilize. The doctor then removes several of the fertilized eggs from the culture dish and inserts them into the woman's uterus, where, everyone hopes, at least one will implant and develop into a fetus.

As you can see, this procedure completely bypasses a woman's fallopian tubes. The eggs move directly from the ovaries to the uterus by way of a culture dish. This is wonderful news for women who have severely damaged fallopian tubes, and who never had any hope of an egg reaching the uterus, much less being fertilized. And that's the group of women for whom this procedure was developed. Using IVF, all a woman needs are functioning ovaries and a normal uterus to become pregnant. The entire IVF procedure is performed on an outpatient basis. It requires a minor surgical procedure, and, for the most part, causes little pain or discomfort. But it does require a substantial investment of time, money, and emotion.

To understand IVF, you first need a better knowledge of the procedure itself. If you eventually elect to undergo IVF, you'd start off by taking medications to stimulate your ovaries to produce several eggs during one cycle. Typically, women preparing to undergo IVF receive Pergonal; therefore, the regimen for this portion of the procedure is the same as what was described for Pergonal therapy earlier in this chapter. You'd take the same drug, and, just like with regular Pergonal therapy, the doctor would monitor the state of your ovaries through ultrasounds and blood tests.

As a general rule, women who respond well to Pergonal and produce a number of eggs are more likely to have a successful procedure than are women whose ovaries can only manage to produce a couple of eggs despite Pergonal's prodding. The most obvious reason for this is that the more eggs produced, the more eggs are available for fertilization. But more than that, an abundance of eggs—at least up to a point—reflects ovaries that are healthy and functioning. When an ovary has to struggle and then barely meets the quota, the eggs are more likely to be of poor quality and thus less likely to fertilize. As a woman ages, it gets harder and harder for her ovaries to produce a large number of ripe, healthy eggs in response to drug stimulation.

At any rate, once the Pergonal caused several eggs to mature, and caused your estrogen level to reach a certain point, you'd stop the Pergonal and instead receive an injection of HCG, the same as with regular Pergonal therapy. In this instance, though, the main purpose of the drug would not be to cause ovulation, but to cause the eggs to undergo the final finishing changes necessary for fertilization. Of course, HCG also causes ovulation within 36 to 48 hours of injection, which isn't something you want to occur with IVF. Once the eggs left the ovary, they'd be lost to retrieval. Therefore, exactly 34 to 36 hours after receiving HCG, you'd report to the hospital or clinic so that the doctor could snatch the ripe eggs from the ovaries before they had a chance to break free of their own accord. Sometime before this happened, your partner would have furnished the hospital laboratory with a semen sample, which the lab would then wash and prepare for insemination.

At times, a doctor may have to use a laparoscope to remove the eggs, although this usually isn't necessary. The most common method for retrieving eggs today is through the use of an ultrasound-guided needle. Using ultrasound to visualize your ovaries, the doctor would insert a needle that's attached to a catheter through your vagina and directly into the ripe follicles on your ovaries. As soon as the needle pierced the follicle, a suction apparatus would suck the egg and follicular fluid through the needle and into a prewarmed test tube. The doctor would repeat this procedure for each and every follicle. The eggs would then be placed in a special solution for a few hours to allow them to mature just a bit more before adding your partner's sperm. This egg and sperm mixture would then be placed in an incubator so that fertilization could occur.

Once the eggs had been retrieved, you'd be free to go home. The egg retrieval process itself may be slightly painful, requiring a light anesthesia, but after it's over, you should feel only minimal discomfort. After the procedure, you'd begin taking progesterone supplements, either through injections or vaginal suppositories, to make sure your endometrium was in prime shape for receiving the eggs once they were fertilized.

For the next couple of days, your eggs and your partner's sperm would mingle in an environment that is precisely controlled for temperature, pH, and oxygen and carbon dioxide concentration. After the eggs and sperm had been together about 16 hours, an embryologist or a specially trained lab technician would carefully check each embryo to see if it had been fertilized and, if so, if it was developing normally. The embryologist would then transfer the normal embryos into a second solution that would allow the embryos to continue to develop. After another day or so, the technician would again check the embryos. If at least some of the eggs had developed normally, you'd report back to the hospital to have them transferred to your uterus. Most doctors won't transfer more than about four embryos at any one time so as not to dramatically increase the risk for a multiple pregnancy. If more than four eggs fertilized, the lab could freeze the extras—a process called cryopreservation—so that they'd be available for transferral to your uterus at a later date.

Now for the really tricky part: getting the eggs to implant in your uterus. To give you a clue as to just how tricky it is, consider this: although 70% to 80% of the eggs retrieved for IVF fertilize, only about 20% of those implant in the uterus.[21] The chance of implantation depends on the quality of the embryo as well as the receptivity of the endometrium. That's why doctors transfer more than one embryo to the uterus at a time—to increase the chances that at least one egg will implant and develop into a fetus.

To have the embryos inserted into your uterus, you'd report to the clinic or hospital. There, you'd lie down on an examination table with your feet in stirrups as if for a pelvic examination. Then, using a special catheter, the doctor would very gently pick up the most viable-looking embryos. The embryos would then be immersed in a special solution designed to make them sticky, thus increasing the chance that they'd cling to the endometrium when they made contact.[22] When everything is ready, the doctor would slide the catheter into your vagina, through your cervix, and into your uterus. During the process, he would be very careful not to touch the endometrium with the catheter; doing so for just an instant could irritate the endometrium, possibly causing it to reject the newly arriving embryos. With the catheter in place, the doctor would then very gently inject the contents of the catheter into the uterus.

To allow the eggs time to nestle into the endometrium, you'd remain lying down, with your head lower than the rest of your body, for the next 2 to 4 hours. After that, you'd be free to go home, but you'd need to keep your activities minimal for the next 24 to 48 hours. After that, you could resume your normal, daily routine—within limits, of course. You'd still want to keep your stress level at a minimum and refrain from heavy lifting or anything that could cause you to overheat, such as vigorous exercise.

After about two weeks, you'd visit your doctor's office for a pregnancy test to see if the procedure was successful. If it wasn't, you'd probably have to wait about two months before attempting IVF a second time.

Figuring out your chances for success with IVF isn't easy. The statistics vary according to who you listen to. Each doctor and each IVF clinic can mean something different when it says that a procedure was "successful." While most women define "success" as going home with a baby, many clinics say that a procedure was successful if a pregnancy resulted. It's important to realize that a pregnancy doesn't necessarily mean a live birth, especially if the pregnancy was a result of IVF. In fact, the pregnancy loss rate following IVF ranges from 30% to 60%. This range is so broad because the simple definition of when a woman is pregnant can vary from clinic to clinic. Some clinics count an IVF procedure a success if a chemical pregnancy results; this is a pregnancy based on a blood test as early as 10 days after implantation that shows a mildly elevated level of HCG. Other than the results of this lab test, a woman would have no inkling that she's pregnant. This is extremely early and, as you may guess, the failure rate of such chemical pregnancies is very high. However, by counting chemical pregnancies, a clinic can increase its number of "successes." Other clinics use what's known as a clinical pregnancy as a marker for success. A clinical pregnancy is when a pregnancy test shows a much higher level of HCG or when an ultrasound shows an embryo with a fetal heartbeat.

But the discrepancies don't end with a clinic's definition of pregnancy. The numbers used to figure success rates—meaning the percentage of women in the program who either became pregnant or delivered babies—also varies widely. Instead of basing their success rate on the total number of women entering an IVF program, many clinics are more selective and completely disregard the number of women who failed to produce enough viable eggs for fertilization. This is significant when you consider that 25% of all women entering such a program won't produce enough eggs. By eliminating these women from their statistics, they can automatically increase their success rate by that much more. Next, some clinics base their success rates on the number of eggs actually retrieved. Still others inflate their success rates even more by only counting the number of eggs that became fertilized.

To help clarify things, consider this situation. You discover an ad in a magazine for an IVF clinic that claims to have an incredible 30% success rate. That sounds encouragingly high to you, so you inquire to find out details. By carefully questioning a doctor at the clinic, you learn that they are counting pregnancy rates and not live births. What's more, out of the 50 women who have entered their program, 13 failed to produce enough eggs for retrieval. That left 37 women. Then, because of premature ovulation or other problems, the doctors failed to retrieve eggs in 6 of the women. Then, of the 31 women who were able to have eggs retrieved, 15 of them failed to have any eggs fertilize.

That left only 16 women who actually had eggs implanted in the uterus. Of these, 5 became pregnant, but only 2 delivered babies. So, if only 2 out of 50 women had babies, how can a clinic claim a 30% success rate? Easy. By defining success as pregnancy—of which there were 5—and basing their success rate on the number of women who had eggs implanted in the uterus—of which there were 16; on that basis, success rate would, indeed, be about 30%. But, if you defined success as a live birth—of which there were 2—and based the success rate on the total number of women entering the program—of which there were 50—then their true "success" rate would only be a measly 4%.

This is a hypothetical situation, but it gives you an idea as to how a clinic's "success" rate can be manipulated. Even renowned fertility specialists hold different opinions on whether they should base their success rates on the total number of women entering the IVF program or on only the number of women who had eggs recovered and placed in a culture dish. Most doctors base their rates on the number of women who had eggs retrieved; but, most women would probably agree that their emotional, not to mention their financial, investment in IVF begins when they start the intensive process to stimulate their ovaries.

Another example of how success rates can be skewed comes from one of the founders of IVF himself, Dr. Patrick Steptoe. In 1989, Dr. Steptoe filed a report based on a review of 1000 babies who were born at his IVF clinic in England since 1978. He reported that, based on the number of women who have had an embryo transferred to the uterus, he had achieved a pregnancy rate of 19%. But, after he subtracted for the number of women who didn't stimulate to make eggs, the women who didn't have an egg fertilized, and the women who had a pregnancy end in miscarriage, he found that the true pregnancy rate per cycle was only 8%.[23]

According to Dr. Gary Ellis of the Office of Technology Assessment, that figure is right on target. In 1989, he testified before a House of Representatives subcommittee that, based on data compiled by IVF clinics for the years 1987 and 1988, a couple had only a 9% chance of taking home a baby after one IVF cycle.[24] Phrased another way, nine out of every ten attempts at IVF end in failure. The chance for a successful IVF pregnancy grows even less with age until, by the time a woman is approaching age 40, it is incredibly slim.

In one study of over 2500 women undergoing IVF during a two-year period, the pregnancy rate for women over age 40 was a scant 6% while the miscarriage rate was an astounding 83%.[25] Out of 94 women of this age group undergoing IVF, only one delivered a baby. According to the scientists, it's difficult to justify continued treatment of patients who have reached age 41. To quote them, "They [women over age 40] have a poor chance of becoming pregnant and very little chance of a pregnancy proceeding to viability."

While these scientists feel that the cutoff point for IVF should be around age 41, other scientists feel that it should come several years earlier, around age 37. To be specific, a study of over 5500 IVF attempts performed in several different clinics in France in 1986 also showed that a woman's age was an indicator as to whether IVF would be successful. The pregnancy rate per attempt fell from 19.8% for women younger than age 25 to no more than 9% for women older than age 40. (These researchers noted that the pregnancy rates reported in this study were somewhat higher than pregnancy rates reported by other researchers because some of the clinics involved in the study included chemical pregnancies in their statistics, which would inflate their success rates, while other clinics counted only clinical pregnancies.) At any rate, when they further analyzed the figures according to the women's ages, they found that the chances for achieving a pregnancy with IVF dropped markedly for women older than age 36. As a result, they concluded that women age 37 or older should be discouraged from trying to attempt pregnancy through IVF.[26]

As with so many other factors of infertility, the reason for this reduction isn't crystal clear. Many scientists say that older women tend to produce fewer eggs in response to ovarian stimulation, and that they also have a slightly greater chance of producing embryos with genetic abnormalities.[27] Others have found that the eggs produced by older women aren't as likely to be fertilized as are the eggs produced by younger women.[28] Still others have claimed that women older than age 35 may produce as many eggs as younger women, and that the eggs may be fertilized, but that, once fertilized, they're less likely to develop normally.[29] Another area that many researchers agree is a significant contributor to an older woman's high risk for a failed IVF procedure is the state of her endometrium.[30–32] They feel that, with age, the endometrium becomes less receptive to the intrusion of a fertilized egg, and that it's no longer up to the heavy responsibility of nourishing and housing this demanding visitor. The reasons for the endometrium's failure could be because fibroids are disrupting the smooth uterine surface; it could also be because the endometrium is thin and weak rather than thick and lush, whether because of a hormonal imbalance or because of a lack of blood supply to the uterine lining. On the other hand, recent studies involving ovum donation suggest that, as long as a woman receives supplements of hormones to boost endometrial development, the age of her endometrium may not be a barrier to supporting a growing embryo. (Ovum donation is discussed in detail later in this chapter.) For now, there aren't any studies on humans that can prove that the endometrium is responsible for the failure of many IVF pregnancies to continue to term. However, studies on animals have shown that, with age, the endometrial lining becomes less receptive to estrogen and progesterone. This alone gives some credence to the scientists' theories that the endometrium may play a role.

What you should conclude from all of this is that, if you feel you may have damaged fallopian tubes, and that you may eventually have to resort to IVF to become pregnant, you shouldn't postpone childbearing for long—at least, that is, if becoming pregnant is important to you. The very best candidates for IVF are women who are young, who have been pregnant before, whose only hindrance to pregnancy is tubal disease, and who respond optimally to the fertility drugs. Even then, the clinical pregnancy rate is about 20%.[33] What all of these statistics boil down to is that it will most likely take more than one IVF procedure before pregnancy results. A real drawback to this, though, is the cost. A single attempt of IVF will cost you anywhere from $6000 to $10,000.

Because IVF is so expensive, and the chances for success so slight, you'd want to make sure you had the procedure performed at the best clinic possible. But choosing a doctor or clinic to perform this procedure can be difficult. Beware: not all clinics are the same. In fact, there can be drastic differences between the success rates of various clinics, but you'd never know it by their advertising.

To begin with, as we discussed earlier, the success rates of clinics can vary wildly depending on how the clinic defines success and on what they're basing their figures. Some clinics have been so creative with their figures that they're able to advertise success rates of as high as 30% and yet they've *never had a live birth*. Although it may seem inconceivable, many clinics have done just that. The government doesn't regulate these ads, so there's nothing—other than ethics—to stop a clinic from misleading women in this way. While an IVF clinic may be interested in helping you have a baby, you need to realize that many clinics are for-profit corporations with stockholders whose overriding interest is simply to make money. Not all IVF clinics are like this, of course, but enough of them are that you need to be careful.

Your first resource for finding a specialist or clinic who is proficient in IVF technology might be your current fertility specialist. If your doctor doesn't perform IVF himself, he might be able to recommend someone who does. Also, even if he does perform the procedure, you'll want to ask specific questions. First, how many of these procedures does he perform a year? (The American Fertility Society recommends that, to retain the proficiency such an exacting procedure requires, a doctor or clinic needs to perform at least 40 IVF procedures a year. Of course, more than this is desirable.) Next, is the IVF program a member of the Society for Assisted Reproductive Technology, or SART? (This is a good sign that the doctor or IVF clinic is interested in learning about such procedures, but you shouldn't consider such membership an endorsement of the member's expertise. SART does, however, compile statistics from its member clinics, including oocytes (eggs) retrieved, fertilization rate, implantation rate, and live births. You can obtain a copy of their report by contacting the American Fertility Society at 2140 11th Avenue South, Suite 200, Birmingham, AL 35205–2800.) Finally, ask how many IVF attempts end in live births. Be specific here, and don't get thrown off course by the term "success rate." Press if you have to to learn on what they're basing their success rate.

While knowing a doctor's or clinic's pregnancy rate can help guide your selection of where to go for IVF, it can't be the sole criterion on which you base your decision. Some doctors or clinics take on more "challenging" cases, such as women older than age 35, women who produce few eggs in response to ovarian stimulation, and men who have poor-quality sperm. For these clinics, the pregnancy rates would be lower, but the clinics might be extremely proficient at performing the procedure. On the other hand, some clinics screen their patients, selecting only those most likely to conceive, so that their pregnancy rates are higher. For these reasons, you should also quiz the doctor or clinic about their experience with patients with your background. For example, if you're over age 35 with endometriosis, ask them about their birth rates for women in your age group with your diagnosis.

Also, besides considering the doctor's ability, you'd want to know something about the laboratory. That's another reason why you want to go somewhere that performs hundreds of these procedures a year as opposed to a few dozen. Keeping eggs and sperm alive in the laboratory requires expert skill and up-to-date equipment. The temperature and pH of the eggs' surroundings must remain constant, and none of the culture medium can evaporate if the egg is to survive. Furthermore, if the egg is left outside the cozy confines of the incubator for more than a couple of minutes, it will die. As you can see, all it takes is a little bit of carelessness on the part of an undertrained lab technician to cause your eggs to die, and, with them, your hopes for a pregnancy.

Many of the success rates cited in this section are from 1987 and 1988, which was several years ago. The reason for this is that there is a lag time of several years between when the procedures are performed and the statistics are compiled, analyzed, and reported. Some doctors feel that the overall success rate of IVF today may be slightly higher than the statistics reported here. The reason, they claim, is that they're becoming more adept: they're better able to stimulate the ovaries to produce eggs; they're becoming more proficient at retrieving and transferring eggs; and they've improved the techniques used to prepare sperm for insemination. But it's going to be difficult for success rates to take much of a leap until research in this area improves.

Research on the IVF procedure has been at a standstill in the United States since about 1980. This occurred because the government became concerned that IVF might be considered unethical. Then, also in 1980, the Department of Health and Human Services—the department responsible for funding grants for medical research—let its Ethics Advisory Board lapse. The sole purpose of the Ethics Advisory Board was to advise the Department of Health and Human Services which research programs were ethical and therefore deserving of funding. So, because the Ethics Advisory Board no longer exists, there isn't anyone to reassure the Department of Health and Human Services that IVF is ethical and that it deserves research support. As a result, no grants requesting money for IVF research are funded. The only research being performed in the United States on the new reproductive technologies are funded solely through private means. Private funding is something, of course, but expansive research projects require large sums of money that only the federal government can provide.

So there you have it—all of the whys and what-fors of IVF. IVF has a fairly low live birth rate, to be sure; that's why it's considered a treatment of last resort. But, for women who have hopelessly damaged fallopian tubes, IVF may be their only chance for becoming pregnant.

Gamete Intrafallopian Transfer

Of course, there are many women who have intact, functioning fallopian tubes but who still can't seem to get pregnant through conventional therapies. Is IVF their only option, too? Fortunately, no. If your fallopian tubes are functioning, a more desirable option would be a variation of IVF called gamete intrafallopian transfer, or GIFT.

GIFT was developed in 1984 by Dr. Ricardo H. Asch, now the director of the Center for Reproductive Health Care at the University of California in Irvine. Dr. Asch had a theory that in many cases of unexplained infertility, pregnancy wasn't occurring because the egg and sperm just weren't meeting in the fallopian tube like they were supposed to. Working with that thought as a premise, Dr. Asch developed GIFT, a procedure in which the doctor takes several eggs from the woman, sperm from her partner, and places both inside the woman's fallopian tube at the same time. This sets the stage for fertilization by making sure that all necessary parties are in the right place at the right time. What results is a pregnancy rate that is significantly higher than the pregnancy rate for IVF.

The GIFT procedure—which costs in the neighborhood of $6000 to $8000—starts out the same as IVF. You'd first receive drugs to stimulate your ovaries to produce multiple follicles, and the status of your ovaries would be closely monitored through daily ultrasounds and blood tests. Then, when the follicles looked fully mature, you'd receive a shot of HCG, just as you would before IVF. Within 36 hours, you'd report to the hospital to have the GIFT procedure performed. Before the scheduled procedure, your partner would have provided the laboratory with a sample of his semen.

Once you arrived at the hospital, you would be placed under general anesthesia in preparation for a laparoscopy. The first step in GIFT is the retrieval of the eggs. The doctor would either do this during the laparoscopy, or he might choose to retrieve the eggs before the laparoscopy by inserting an ultrasound-guided needle through the vagina and into the follicles, just as would be done for IVF. Regardless of how they're obtained, once the eggs are outside your body, an embryologist would immediately examine them under a microscope, judging each for its quality and level of development. Depending upon how many mature eggs were available, the doctor would load two to four of them into a catheter along with a sample of your partner's sperm. When filling the catheter, the doctor would make sure that a small bead of air separated the sperm from the eggs. This way, he could be sure that fertilization would only occur inside the fallopian tube and not inside the catheter.

The doctor would then use the laparoscope to locate the open end of the fallopian tube closest to the ovary. Once he isolated this tiny target, the doctor would slide the catheter about an inch or so inside the fallopian tube and then gently inject the eggs and sperm. Typically, doctors inject two eggs and some sperm in one fallopian tube, and another two eggs and sperm in the other tube. That's all there is to it. The entire procedure takes only 45 minutes to an hour. After you'd recovered from the anesthesia, you'd be free to return home. You'd need to remain sedentary for a day or so, but, after that, you could resume your normal activities. However, you'd want to avoid doing anything strenuous, or anything that would raise your body's temperature, until you learned whether or not you were pregnant.

An advantage of GIFT is that it allows egg and sperm to meet inside their own territory, the fallopian tube. Besides the advantage of residing in their own temperature- and pH-controlled environment, becoming fertilized in the fallopian tube allows the embryo to move to the uterus at its own pace, implanting according to nature's timetable and not the laboratory's. Under normal conditions, the embryo travels down the fallopian tube for several days and then floats in the uterus for a couple of more days before ever implanting. Therefore, the embryo is close to a week old before it ever burrows into the endometrium. This is in stark contrast to IVF, in which the embryo is transferred to the uterus when it is only a couple of days old. But, because it would be extremely difficult to keep an embryo alive for that long in a laboratory, there really is no other choice. Another advantage of GIFT is that the embryo can drop out of the fallopian tube and sink into the endometrium of its own accord. This is, obviously, much gentler than being projected out of the end of a syringe.

All of these factors have no doubt helped to bolster GIFT's pregnancy rate, making it about twice as high as for IVF. According to one expert, after subtracting for miscarriages and pregnancies that didn't develop, the pregnancy rate after 1156 GIFT cycles was 21.3%.[34] As you can see, that's much better than the 9% overall pregnancy rate for IVF. Of course, GIFT has one significant prerequisite, and that's that at least one fallopian tube be open and functioning normally. After all, that's the whole point of GIFT: to deposit the eggs and sperm in the fallopian tube. If a woman's fallopian tubes are scarred closed or otherwise damaged, GIFT isn't an option. In that instance, IVF is the only choice.

While intact fallopian tubes are the only prerequisite to having a GIFT procedure performed, there are several other factors that influence the procedure's outcome. The first such factor is the availability of mature, healthy eggs for transferral. As you know, when the doctor retrieves the eggs, an embryologist immediately examines them, grading each according to its level of maturity. The highest grade an egg can receive is a 5; therefore, an egg that receives a grade of 4+ or 5 is considered extremely mature, a prime candidate for fertilization. The more of these top-quality eggs a woman produces, the better are her chances for pregnancy. In fact, a study of 218 GIFT procedures at two of the top infertility centers in the United States revealed a direct association between the number of quality eggs transferred and the pregnancy rate. For women who didn't produce any eggs that could earn a grade of 4+ or 5, the pregnancy rate following GIFT was only 16.5%. For women who produced and had transferred two eggs with this outstanding grade, the pregnancy rate increased to 25%. Finally, for women who had three or more of these prime eggs available for transfer, the pregnancy rate was an impressive 50%.[35]

Of course, as you age, it's going to become increasingly difficult for your ovaries to muster the energy required to produce such prime eggs. That's one reason why, the older you are, the lower are your chances for having a baby as a result of a GIFT procedure. As a result, some experts have taken the stand that doctors should transfer more than the usual three or four eggs in certain cases, such as when the woman is older or when she has polycystic ovarian disease (a disorder that causes her to produce a large number of suboptimum eggs). The main argument for limiting the number of eggs transferred to three or four is the same one used for IVF: to minimize the risk of multiple pregnancy. (In most GIFT cycles, there's a 30% chance for having twins; in the normal population, the rate is only 1.4%.)[36]

But GIFT is a different procedure than IVF. With GIFT, doctors transfer eggs, not embryos. They have no way of knowing whether any, or all, of the eggs placed inside the fallopian tubes will be fertilized. On the other hand, with IVF, only eggs that have already been fertilized are transferred to the woman's uterus. Of course, GIFT has a much higher implantation rate than does IVF—and that's the main reason doctors have felt that they should continue to limit the number of eggs transferred to the fallopian tubes. But, at least one study has shown that this may not be such a good practice, particularly when dealing with older women.

This study, which involved more than 1000 women, showed that women age 40 or older undergoing a GIFT procedure had to have every egg available (which sometimes totaled 11 or more) transferred to achieve a pregnancy rate of 19.2%.[37] Keep in mind that that's *pregnancy* rate, not *birth* rate. Because the miscarriage rate following GIFT for women age 40 or greater is a depressing 48.6%, the actual birth rate is about half that.[38] What's more, even with transferring this many eggs, the multiple pregnancy rate in this group of women was significantly lower than it was for younger women. This only seems to underscore the point that restricting the number of eggs transferred when a woman's age is an issue hurts more than it helps. Instead of limiting her risk of having more than one baby, the chances are greater that it will keep her from having any baby at all.

Besides the number and quality of eggs transferred, another variable in the success of GIFT is the quality of the sperm. To illustrate how significant sperm quality can be, consider the following study. After performing 218 GIFT cycles, doctors figured that the overall pregnancy rate for the procedure was 28.4%. Then, to try to get a better idea of the true success rate, they separated out all of the cases for which sperm quality was a factor and analyzed them separately. What they discovered was significant. When the sperm used in a GIFT procedure was suboptimal in quality, a woman had only a 6.1% chance of becoming pregnant following a GIFT procedure. But, when sperm quality wasn't a factor, a woman had a very respectable 33% chance of becoming pregnant with GIFT.[39]

The researchers also discovered that the most important aspect of sperm wasn't their number, but rather their shape and how well they moved. To be specific, researchers found that couples who had sperm counts of 20 million or less before the sperm were washed had a pregnancy rate with GIFT that was similar to couples who had much higher sperm counts. However, if 30% or fewer of the sperm moved normally, or if 50% or fewer of the sperm had a normal shape, then pregnancy rates plummeted. To be specific, when *more* than 50% of the sperm were shaped normally, the pregnancy rate from GIFT was about

36%. But, when 50% or fewer of the sperm were shaped normally, the pregnancy rate slipped by two-thirds to less than 11%. Also, when *more* than 30% of the sperm moved well, the pregnancy rate was about 32%. But, when fewer than 30% of the sperm had good motility, the pregnancy rate was slashed by four-fifths to less than 7%.

All in all, though, if your fallopian tubes are intact, if your ovaries can still produce good-quality eggs, and if your partner has a normal semen analysis, then you'd have a decent chance of becoming pregnant through GIFT. Even more good news about GIFT is that it seems to work in women who have untreated endometriosis.

As you may recall, endometriosis can be difficult to treat when pregnancy is the desired goal. Doctors haven't been sure exactly what course of action is the best. But, according to one study, as long as the woman has at least one functioning fallopian tube, her chance of success with GIFT is comparable to the success rates in women who don't have endometriosis.[40] This study analyzed the results of GIFT procedures on 327 women, 46 of whom had endometriosis. The pregnancy rate for all groups of women, regardless of diagnosis, was 23.7%, with an ongoing pregnancy rate of 18.1%. When the researchers analyzed the pregnancy rate for just the women who had endometriosis, they were pleased to discover that it was 30.5%. This is incredibly encouraging, especially considering that no other treatment of endometriosis, when the desired outcome is pregnancy, has had results that are nearly that good.

Again, GIFT is one of the exciting new reproductive technologies. For young women whose ovaries produce multiple, prime eggs, and whose partners have at least normal fertility, the success rate can be quite high. With age, though, the success rate declines. Furthermore, a major drawback with GIFT is that it doesn't answer the question of whether the eggs are actually fertilizable by the male's sperm. This is particularly important if your partner has a poor semen analysis or if he has antisperm antibodies. To counter these shortcomings, doctors devised yet another procedure: zygote intrafallopian transfer, or ZIFT.

Zygote Intrafallopian Transfer

ZIFT is a hybrid of GIFT and IVF, blending the best of both technologies. The ZIFT procedure starts out just like IVF: you'd have your ovaries stimulated to produce multiple eggs, and then the doctor would retrieve the mature eggs through the use of an ultrasound-guided needle inserted through the vagina. Then, again just as with IVF, the eggs would be placed in a culture medium with a sample of your partner's sperm for fertilization. The mixture would be placed in an incubator for a couple of days and you would go home.

Now, this is where the procedure differs from IVF. Once the eggs had fertilized, you'd report to the hospital to have them transferred to your fallopian tubes, not your uterus. Of course, this step of the procedure involves a laparoscopy, just like with GIFT. The only difference here is that the doctor would be transferring eggs that were already fertilized (called zygotes). These fertilized eggs, once they entered the fallopian tubes, would then travel the length of the tube at their own pace, dropping gently down into the endometrium when they're ready.

It's easy to see the benefit of this procedure. Because the doctor is only transferring eggs that have already been fertilized, there isn't any question as to whether fertilization will occur. Also, because the eggs are being inserted into the fallopian tubes instead of the uterus, they have the advantage of settling into the endometrium according to their own timetable, thus improving the implantation rate. The pregnancy rate for ZIFT is about the same as it is for GIFT, except in cases of male infertility, in which cases it's even higher. The one prerequisite, though, just like with GIFT, is that you must have at least one functioning fallopian tube.

A disadvantage of ZIFT is that it requires two separate procedures, one of them surgical. You'd have to have the eggs retrieved, and then, one or two days later, you'd have a laparoscopy to have the fertilized eggs inserted into your fallopian tubes. ZIFT would also be more expensive than either IVF or

GIFT. After all, you'd have to pay the expenses of the embryology lab that would keep your eggs alive—the same expenses that you'd have for IVF—plus you'd have to pay the hospital and doctor fees for a laparoscopy—the same as for a GIFT procedure.

But, if your partner has an abnormal semen analysis—particularly if a significant number of the sperm have an abnormal shape or have poor motility—then ZIFT would give you the best possible odds of achieving pregnancy. Also, ZIFT would be the procedure for you if you had any other reason to suspect that your partner's sperm weren't able to fertilize your eggs, such as if your partner had antisperm antibodies or if you'd had a failed GIFT procedure.

*   *   *

Overall, these IVF technologies, which include GIFT and ZIFT, have allowed doctors to make great strides toward making pregnancy and childbirth possible for a multitude of women who otherwise wouldn't be able to conceive. It also appears that the children conceived through the help of these technologies are no different from children who are conceived naturally.

To date, about 4000 children have been conceived through either IVF or GIFT. These children have no greater incidence of birth defects, and they were just as healthy at birth as was any other child. The only thing that places the child's health at any greater risk is when a multiple pregnancy occurs.

You may think that a 20 to 30% chance of pregnancy doesn't sound very high. But remember, even under ideal circumstances, the chances of pregnancy occurring in any one month is no more than about 30%. Also, compared to IVF or some of the other infertility treatments, these pregnancy rates are quite high, indeed. Of course, age is still a factor. If you postpone parenthood until you're age 40 or so, your chances for success with any one of these procedures will be markedly diminished. That's why, at that point, you may wish to consider oocyte donation.

Oocyte Donation

As we've already discussed, one of the main reasons fertility declines with age is that the quality of the eggs, or oocytes, declines. A fairly new technology that's available to combat that problem is oocyte donation. Essentially, the technique involves retrieving eggs from a younger woman, combining those eggs with your partner's sperm, and then transferring those eggs to your reproductive system. The transferral could occur through either IVF, GIFT, or ZIFT. Then, if all goes well, the embryo would implant in your uterus, and, nine months later, you'd give birth to a child who had half of your husband's genes and half of the genes of the woman donor.

Although oocyte donation procedures have been performed since about 1978, it's only recently received attention as being a possible treatment for older women who haven't been able to conceive through other means. Until now, the procedure was reserved for younger women who experienced premature menopause (before age 30), for women who had no ovaries, or for women who risked transmitting a genetic disease to their offspring. Then, in 1990, a group of doctors from the University of Southern California published a study in the *New England Journal of Medicine* that caused the medical community to look upon this procedure in a new light.[41]

In this study, the doctors retrieved oocytes from three fertile women between the ages of 31 and 34. These eggs were fertilized with the sperm of different men, and the resulting embryos were then transferred to seven women between the ages of 40 and 44 whose ovaries no longer functioned, meaning that they had already gone through menopause. Both before and after receiving the embryos, the women took hormones to prepare and maintain their endometrial linings. The results were amazing. Out of the 28 embryos transferred during eight separate procedures, ten implantations occurred, resulting in an implantation rate of 36%. Out of the seven women, five gave birth to normal, healthy infants. One other woman had a miscarriage, while the last woman had a stillborn infant. What's even more surprising is that, when the doctors compared these results to a control group of younger women undergoing this same procedure, they found no difference in results. This led the doctors to conclude that the main problem older women face when trying to conceive and carry a child to term is the problem of old eggs. They also found that, with proper hormonal support, a woman's endometrium could provide a receptive environment in which an embryo could implant and grow.

When looking at these results, though, you need to keep several factors in mind. To begin with, this was a very small study of only seven women, although other studies have supported these findings. Second, none of the women in the group were older than age 44. And finally, all of the women in this study had stopped ovulating altogether. This means that, for women who are older than age 40 but who still ovulate—even if they do so irregularly—the results may not be as promising. For this reason, women who still ovulate and wish to undergo oocyte donation must take medications to induce temporary "menopause." And finally, the only problem with the women in this study was that they had gone through menopause early. Other women of the same age might have other health problems impinging on their fertility.

Also, while some studies have supported the findings that it's the age of the donor that's important, not the age of the recipient, other studies have not found this to be true. For example, in a study of 82 patients undergoing 100 cycles of oocyte donation, the researchers noted that the age of the donor didn't influence the outcome (although most of the donors were age 35 or younger), but that as the age of the recipient increased, the pregnancy rate decreased.[42] In this instance, the pregnancy rate for women aged 25 to 29 was an impressive 50%; however, the pregnancy rate for women aged 45 to 49 was only 9.7%.

In addition, there are several problems with oocyte donation that you should consider. Besides the cost, which runs about $10,000, it can also be difficult to find a donor. Typically, donors have been women whose ovaries have been stimulated for IVF. If they produce more eggs than they can use, they have the option of donating the extra eggs to an infertile couple. However, now that freezing embryos has become a possibility, most couples choose this option instead. As a result, some clinics have taken to soliciting donors. Most such donors are paid a fee of about $2000; doctors try to keep reimbursement small so that money doesn't become a motivating factor in making the donation.

Most clinics, though, leave it up to the woman receiving the embryo to find the donor. Possible donors include friends and relatives, such as a younger sister or cousin. In these instances, of course, you'd know who the donor was. In all other cases, the donor usually remains anonymous.

The ideal donor is under age 35 and has had as many children as she wants. Besides undergoing a complete medical examination, including screenings for hereditary and sexually transmitted diseases, the donor also undergoes a complete psychological analysis. It's also a good idea to have the donor sign a contract clarifying your arrangement and discussing such matters as the donor's relinquishment of all rights to the offspring and who's responsible if the child has a birth defect.

Once the donor is accepted, she would undergo a cycle of drugs to stimulate her ovaries to produce multiple eggs. The process she would go through would be the same as for routine Pergonal therapy, which was described earlier in the chapter. Once the follicles reached a certain size, the donor would receive a shot of HCG, and then the doctor would retrieve the eggs using ultrasound. Then, depending upon the circumstances, the egg would be immediately transferred to the recipient, or it would be fertilized and then frozen for later implantation.

And therein lies the other problem: synchronizing the cycle of the recipient to that of the donor. As you already know, an embryo can be kept alive in a lab for only so long. Doctors also know that the margin of time in which the endometrium is receptive to the intrusion of an embryo is slight. Although they don't know for sure when the most optimal time is, they've been able to narrow it down to between days 16 and 19. To make sure your endometrium is at that stage at the exact time that the donor's eggs are mature requires some deft hormonal juggling. If your ovaries are still functioning at all—meaning that they're producing at least some amount of hormones on their own—then you'd first have to take certain hormones to override the functions of your ovaries, and then you'd have to take supplements of still other hormones to get you started on a new track. The whole while, the doctor would have to keep in mind the donor's cycle, focusing on when the follicles would be ready for retrieval. If you have already gone through menopause, the doctor would give you hormones to stimulate your endometrium to mature in anticipation of an arriving embryo. Then, once the embryo was transferred to your uterus, you'd continue taking hormone supplements for at least the next couple of weeks and, if pregnancy occurred, you'd continue taking hormones for the next three to four months, or until the placenta could take over the job of supplying all of the necessary hormones.

If you think you might ever be interested in having oocyte donation, you'd need to consider more than just the medical difficulties of such a procedure. There's also the ethical implications to consider.

The American Fertility Society has declared oocyte donation to be an ethically acceptable procedure. It only qualifies its stand by saying that donors should be paid solely for their expenses and their time and inconvenience. But other medical ethicists have a problem with oocyte donation, feeling uncomfortable with the whole idea of "buying" an egg. In addition, there's the possibility of a lawsuit arising at some point in the future over who is the baby's real mother. That hasn't happened yet, but it's bound to at some point.

One reason for this is that egg donation is so much more risky and intrusive than is sperm donation. As a result, a woman donor may feel she has more invested in the process. Also, fewer children are likely to result from a woman's donation—because of the limited supply of eggs—than result from a man's sperm donation, meaning that a woman may feel more "connected" to the eggs she's donated.

From the recipient's standpoint, there are other factors to

consider. To begin with, just as with donor insemination, would you and your partner be able to accept a child as your own who only had your partner's genes along with the genes of another woman? On the positive side, oocyte donation would give you the benefit of carrying the fetus through all of its stages of growth and then actually giving birth yourself.

Even with its difficulties, oocyte donation is becoming increasingly popular. In 1990, 48 medical centers offered egg donor programs. That's up from 26 centers the year before.

Oocyte donation is certainly a real option, and, given the increase in the number of centers offering the service, it appears to be here to stay. While the procedure is certainly available if you suddenly learn that the time on your eggs has expired when you're ready to conceive, it's not a procedure that you'd enter into lightly. Both you and your partner would have to thoroughly evaluate all of the pros and cons of such a procedure before making the choice.

Conclusion

At this point, you may not even know when you want to get pregnant, much less whether or not you'll require medical help to do so. Regardless, now that you know about the types of treatments available, you know there is no such thing as a "miracle cure" for infertility. Be assured, though, that if you find you have a problem becoming pregnant when you decide the time is right, treatments exist that can most likely help you conceive. Keep in mind, though, that most treatments are time-consuming, expensive, emotionally draining—and some have a high degree of failure. In other words, they're not something you want to rely on as insurance. The key, then, is to try to foresee, as much as is humanly possible, whether or not you'll have a problem and then plan accordingly. Doing so now could help you save a lot of time and heartache in the future.

10

Is Adoption an Option?

Throughout your years of postponement, you may be comforting yourself with the thought that, even if you can't have children of your own, you can always adopt. No problem, right? Well, actually, adopting a child isn't as easy as it once was. Couples who face the greatest difficulty are those who wish to adopt a healthy, white infant. In fact, some estimate that about 50 couples want to adopt each white infant who becomes available.[1] The odds are a little better for couples wishing to adopt a child of color; even then, though, it's not as easy as you might think.

One reason for the intense competition for healthy babies is that many women who find themselves saddled with an unwanted pregnancy opt for abortion. In addition, it's become much more socially acceptable for an unmarried woman to give birth to, and then raise, a child by herself. To be specific, about 95% of unmarried mothers now keep their babies instead of giving them up for adoption.[2]

But adoption *is* possible—it's just not easy. To give you some encouragement, you should know that about 50,000 children are adopted each year. Some of these are healthy white infants; others are children of color; still others are older or are from foreign countries. Adoption is an option, to be sure; it's just not an option you can easily latch onto at the last minute. To give yourself the broadest knowledge base possible when making decisions about when, and how, to start your family, you owe it to yourself to learn a little bit about the adoption process.

The Adoption Myth

Before going any further, we need to take a minute and debunk one of the most popular myths concerning adoption, and that's that adoption can help "cure" infertility. Almost everyone has heard stories about couples who tried and tried without success to have a baby only to become pregnant shortly after adopting. Adoption relieved the pressure to have a child, people have reasoned, and thus allowed the couple to conceive a baby of their own. You need to know that, for the most part, this just isn't true. Sure, some couples conceive after adopting a child, but they are definitely in the minority. One study of 100 adopting couples found that this occurred only 4% of the time.[3] You stand to gain many things by adopting a child, but conceiving a child of your own isn't likely to be one of them.

Adoption Options

There are three basic ways of adopting a child. The first way is the traditional way and involves working with an agency that matches available children with suitable couples. A second way, which is becoming increasingly popular, bypasses agencies and instead enlists the aid of an attorney to arrange the adoption privately, or independently. And finally, a third option many couples are choosing is to adopt a child from a foreign county.

Agency Adoption

Agency adoption is the type of adoption with which most people are familiar. The agency acts as an intermediary between the birth mother and the adoptive couple, working to place the child in the best environment possible. An agency adoption is typically a safe adoption; agencies take care of all of the necessary legal work and wait to place a child until any possible loophole has been closed.

Two kinds of adoption agencies exist: public and private. Most couples wishing to adopt an infant today choose to work with private agencies, probably because public agencies tend to have very few infants available for adoption. One reason for this is that, as state-run institutions, public agencies have a kind of stigma attached to them that most unmarried, pregnant women wish to avoid. As a result, if a woman has a baby she wants to give up for adoption, she'll most likely seek out a private agency to handle the matter. Public agencies aren't all bad, though. A big advantage is that adoptions handled through public agencies are inexpensive. The city or state pays all of the biological mother's medical and legal costs, which is the bulk of the expense in any adoption. Private agencies, on the other hand, ask the adopting couple to pay all of the birth mother's medical expenses that aren't covered by insurance, her legal costs, and perhaps some of her housing expenses until the baby is born. This can add up quickly. In fact, according to the National Committee for Adoption, the average cost of a domestic adoption through an agency in 1989 was about $14,500.[4]

Now, let me quickly say this doesn't mean that, under every circumstance, you'd have to *pay* that much to adopt. Some agencies, particularly those specializing in the adoption of children with special needs, charge significantly less and then make up the difference through fund raising or outside contributions. Just be aware: adoptions can be quite expensive. In fact, some agencies charge couples as much as $30,000 to adopt.

With all that said, you need to know that the expense of adoption may not be the worst part—at least, that is, if you want to adopt a baby. Even at private agencies, infants are in incredibly short supply. Couples who want to adopt a newborn typically have to wait from three to six years before receiving a call that a baby is available. And, because agencies don't want the waiting period to grow even longer, they work at limiting the number of people on their waiting lists.

One way they do this is by discouraging people making telephone inquiries about adopting a baby. For example, if you call an agency and say you're interested in adopting a baby, you're likely to be told that they're not accepting applications for infant adoptions and that they are, instead, concentrating on placing older children and children with handicaps. This may very well be true, but you can't just accept this news and hang up. You have to press. Ask *when* they'll be accepting applications. Some agencies accept applications only at certain times of the year. Another tactic is to ask if the agency conducts orientation meetings for prospective adoptive parents. If so, tell them you'd like to attend.

Most agencies do conduct such meetings. These meetings usually consist of a social worker addressing a group of couples interested in adoption, informing them of the agency's procedures, fees, and requirements. During these meetings, the social workers typically spend at least a portion of the time emphasizing the shortage of infants. They usually try to encourage the couples present to consider adopting an older child or a child with special needs instead of a baby. If this option appeals to you, that's wonderful. But if it doesn't, don't feel you have to give up on your idea of a baby. Just listening to all the social worker has to say will tell you a lot about the qualities the agency looks for in prospective parents. After all, if you want to adopt, you'd have to convince the agency that you and your partner would make ideal parents, and to do that, you'd need to know what they expect. Sure, you may know that you and your partner would be perfect parents, but the agencies have the children. You'd have to convince them.

After the social worker finished speaking, you'd be invited to fill out a short application form and arrange an appointment for a personal meeting with a social worker. This meeting is the first, crucial step in the adoption process. Some agencies exclude couples based on their application and this first interview alone. Therefore, you and your partner would need to be prepared. You should discuss every possible aspect of adoption with each other before the interview. Why do you want to adopt a child? Would you consider an older child or a child with special needs? How do you think your family and friends will respond to your decision to adopt? You'd want to explore these issues thoroughly so that you and your partner could exude confidence and calmness during the interview; you'd want there to be no doubt in the social worker's mind that you'd make good parents.

During the interview, the social worker would gather biographical data, such as your ages and how long you'd been married, and she'd also delve into more personal issues, such as your reasons for adopting and what kind of child you wished to adopt. She may also ask whether you've consulted with any other agencies. Be forewarned that some agencies require a couple to work with it exclusively. From the agency's point of view, they're devoting time and energy to helping you find a child, and they don't want that time to be wasted if you decide to adopt elsewhere. But, from your point of view, if you limit yourself to one agency, you'd also be limiting your chances for finding a baby. If you do choose to work with more than one agency at a time, you'd need to be discreet.

During the interview, the social worker would also work at gathering information to help determine whether you fit the profile of what the agency thinks adoptive parents should be like. Some of this will be based on subjective data, such as how the social worker feels about you. In addition to this, though, the agency has certain criteria that you'd be expected to meet.

To begin with, most agencies have a policy of not accepting applicants over a certain age. Although the agency may not admit this to you, you can be assured that they *do* use age as a criterion. The usual cutoff for someone wishing to adopt an infant is age 40, although some agencies won't accept anyone over the age of 35. Even if you want to adopt an older child, most agencies don't want you to be more than 40 years older than the child.

Also, most agencies won't accept a couple who isn't married. What's more, how long you've been married could also influence the agency's decision. If you've only been married a short time, the social worker could feel that enough time hadn't passed to determine whether your marriage is stable. At the other extreme, if you've been married for a number of years—say, ten years—without having children, the social worker could surmise that children really aren't that important to you. Furthermore, how many times you've been married could influence her decision. For example, if you've been married four times and divorced three, the social worker could question whether you'd be an ideal candidate to receive a child.

Next, the agency would want to make sure that you and your spouse had good, stable jobs and that you made enough money to support a child. This involves inquiring about your educational backgrounds and job histories. The agency would also want details about your finances, including specifics regarding your savings accounts, investments, any property you owned (such as your house), as well as any debts. They'd also want to know what kind of life and health insurance policies you have.

After this, they'd want more personal information about you—such as, are you mentally and physically healthy? Some agencies have rules against placing children with couples who are grossly overweight or who smoke. To attest to the state of your health, you'd probably have to have your and your partner's doctors write a letter to the agency. Also, because most agencies won't allow a couple who can have children of their own adopt a baby, they'd probably want to see records pertaining to your infertility. By doing so, they could learn firsthand whether or not you can have children on your own and whether you'd exhausted all reasonable medical remedies before pursuing adoption.

This may seem intrusive so far, but brace yourself. Most

agencies would also want the woman to make a statement that she'd quit her job and stay home to care for the child if they were allowed to adopt. Yes, that may seem unfair, but it may help if you consider the agency's position. With so many couples vying for so few infants, agencies feel justified in rejecting a couple who plan to put their adopted child in day-care.

When the interview is finally over, you'd go home and the social worker would write a report recommending whether or not the agency should accept your application. If you were to be rejected, you'd receive a form letter notifying you of that fact. Of course, this wouldn't tell you why you were rejected. You'd probably never learn that. Even calling the agency probably wouldn't produce any details. The reason for your rejection could be an extremely small one. Maybe it was your age, or maybe the social worker felt that you were being too restrictive about the type of child you wanted to adopt. Who knows? Regardless, being rejected doesn't mean that you and your partner wouldn't make good parents. Remember that agencies work at limiting the number of couples on their waiting lists. This means eliminating more applicants than they accept.

But, if the social worker felt that you satisfied all of the agency's requirements for adoptive parents, you'd receive a letter notifying you of this and inviting you to complete a longer application form. With this, the agency may request certain documents, such as marriage and birth certificates, divorce decrees, financial statements, insurance policies, medical reports, as well as letters of recommendation from people vouching for your character. They'd also do a background check to make sure that you and your partner didn't have a criminal record and that you'd never been charged with child abuse. This is also the time that you'd arrange for a home study. Both the long application and the home study aren't free. You'd have to pay for this part of the adoption up-front. How much this costs varies from agency to agency, so it may be worthwhile to inquire about these fees ahead of time. On average, though, the home study will cost about $500 or $600.

The home study isn't just one interview. It's actually an intensive process that involves three interviews with a social worker: one for you alone, one for your spouse alone, and one for both of you together in your home. This time, the social worker would delve even deeper into the relationship between you and your partner. She'd want to know how you felt about parenting, your family, your marriage, and your career. Again, you may resent having to prove to someone you don't even know that you'd make a good parent, but, unfortunately, the agency has the upper hand. So bear with it and, hopefully, a short time after completing the home study, you'd receive a letter from the agency telling you that you had been accepted for placement of an infant. That's great news; no doubt about it. But then you'd have to deal with what may be the hardest part of all: the waiting.

Exactly when you'd receive your child is impossible to answer. It could be one year, or it could be six. The waiting list for a baby isn't like any other waiting list. You'd never know when you'd be "next." Part of the reason for this is that agencies have always tried hard to "match" infants to parents, considering perhaps certain background information or even, at times, trying to match certain physical qualities between the birth and adoptive parents. But, with the shortage of infants, things have changed, mostly in the fact that birth mothers have much more of a say in who adopts their babies. A birth mother may look through several applications and résumés of couples wanting to adopt, searching for a couple with whom she feels comfortable. Depending on the agency, the birth mother may even ask to meet some of the couples before making her decision.

Many couples seeking to adopt are naturally hesitant to meet the birth mother. Some people think they'll feel awkward, or even jealous of the fact that they'll be meeting someone who can do what they can't—which is get pregnant. However, in the end, most couples feel that such a meeting has a very positive effect. If you end up adopting this woman's child, meeting her could be a great opportunity. Besides allowing you to know something about the mother and perhaps setting your mind at ease, it would also give you something to tell your child when he asks questions about where he came from. In addition, meeting the birth mother would give you the chance to reassure her that you'd love and care for her baby if given the chance to adopt. In short, it could help you swing her decision in your favor.

Whether you were to meet the birth mother or not—and many couples never do—the day would eventually come when you'd receive a call that the adoption agency had a baby they wanted to place with you. This is what you would have been waiting for. Finally you'd be a parent. But, even though you'd have a baby in your arms, the procedure wouldn't be over. You'd still have to go through the legal process of making the baby your own.

Your first step in this final journey would be to sign certain documents stating your intention to adopt. Also, before you'd even received the baby, the birth mother would have signed documents surrendering the baby to you. The birth mother would also need to sign still more documents terminating her rights to the baby. When she'd do this would depend upon the rules of your state. Some states allow the birth mother to sign relinquishment papers immediately after birth, while others require a wait of up to 15 days. You also need to know that the decision to give up a child for adoption is often not the mother's to make alone. In most states, the putative father must also sign documents relinquishing his rights to the baby.

Even after all of these documents are signed, the adoption still wouldn't be final. You'd then have to wait through a probationary period during which the social worker would periodically check with you to see how you were functioning in your new role as a parent. How long this probationary period would last depends upon your state's laws, but, in most states, it lasts six months. When those months were over, though, you'd be almost home free. The final step would be to go to court to make the adoption final. However, you just can't show up at the courthouse. You'd first have to submit a ream of documents that makes your tax return look like child's play. To give you some idea of the legal complexities involved, the documents you'd have to submit would include a petition of adoption, an agreement of adoption, an affidavit that detailed the financial aspects of the adoption, an affidavit of marriage, an affidavit of medical history of the child, and a notification of the order of adoption. As you can see, this isn't a simple process. Many couples retain their own attorney just to have someone double-check and make sure that all of the documents have been properly executed. The one document you'd want to be absolutely certain had been completed and filed appropriately is the biological mother's surrender statement. One slipup here and the adoption might not be valid, meaning that the birth mother could conceivably try to reclaim her child at a later date.

This would be an unusual occurrence, though, and the odds are good that everything would progress as planned. If so, six months to a year from the time you first received your baby, you'd go to court to make the adoption final. Finally, the baby would be all yours. A few weeks later, you'd receive a new birth certificate for your baby listing you and your partner as the parents. The old birth records would then be sealed along with the adoption records.

Needless to say, adoption is not a simple process. That's where working with an agency can prove advantageous. Agencies are familiar with the ins and outs of adoption law, and they make sure that all of the legal forms are completed and filed as required. Another advantage of agencies is that they strive to make the adoption work. Most even provide counseling services for the biological parents, which can help resolve any conflicts ahead of time, making the actual adoption process much smoother. And finally, agency adoptions are safer for you. Because most agencies won't place an infant with an adopting couple until the birth parents have signed the papers relinquishing their rights to the child, you're protected from the birth mother changing her mind at the last minute.

But, despite these obvious advantages, agencies have some big disadvantages. First, there's the waiting time. Waiting five years to receive an infant is intolerable to many couples, especially couples who have postponed beginning a family. Also, there's the agencies' restrictive criteria to consider. You may not qualify for a child because of any one of a number of reasons, not the least of which is age. So, for these reasons and more, many couples today are choosing to skip agencies altogether and adopt privately.

Private Adoptions

Private, or independent, adoptions bypass the agencies almost entirely. In these adoptions, a couple searches for a pregnant woman who wants to give up her baby for adoption and then works with the birth mother—either personally or through an intermediary—to bring the adoption to a close. Certain couples make the choice to adopt privately because they want to adopt a healthy newborn and they don't want to wait two to six years to do so. Other couples make this choice because they can't meet the strict criteria set by adoption agencies. For example, a couple may be considered "too old" by agency standards. Many people prefer private adoptions because they are actively involved in the process instead of being forced to sit back and wait while an agency calls the shots. Be forewarned, though, that private adoptions are riskier than are adoptions through an agency. There's a much greater chance that the adoption will fail, leaving you emotionally drained and, perhaps, financially depleted.

But, before getting into those issues, you need to understand how a private adoption works. Let's say you want to adopt privately. How would you go about it? Your first—and perhaps most essential—step would be to consult a good lawyer specializing in adoption. The laws regarding private adoption vary tremendously from state to state, and you need to have someone in the know guiding you.

One of the best ways to find such a lawyer would be by a referral from a couple who had successfully completed a private adoption. How do you find such couples? By simply talking to people. Join an adoption support group, whether through Resolve or one of the other groups listed in Appendix B. Besides being able to advise you about lawyers, such groups can provide you with a wealth of other information about adoptions in your area. You should also visit your library or local bookstore for books on adoption. Not only will these books bring you up-to-date on the intricacies of private adoption, you might also uncover the name of a lawyer who would be just right for you. And finally, you could look in the yellow pages of your telephone book or call the local chapter of the American Bar Association for the names of adoption lawyers in your area. Once you had a list of names, you'd begin calling each lawyer's office, searching for the lawyer who had handled the most successful adoptions. It would also be important to make sure that the lawyer you selected was familiar with both state and federal laws regarding adoption.

A good lawyer can be the key to a successful adoption. Besides helping you make sure all necessary documents are completed and filed appropriately, a lawyer can inform you what your state will or won't permit with regard to arranging an adoption. For example, some states won't allow a third party, such as a doctor or a lawyer, to bring adoptive and birth parents together. Other states won't allow couples to advertise their desire to meet a woman willing to give up her infant for adoption. And finally, some states have outlawed independent adoption altogether. These states include Connecticut, Delaware, Massachusetts, Michigan, Minnesota, and North Dakota. (However, in Connecticut, Massachusetts, and North Dakota, couples are allowed to find birth mothers on their own; they just have to complete the adoption process through an agency instead of through a lawyer. In the other states, adopting independently simply isn't an option.)

Now, don't get the wrong idea about private adoptions just

because some states have declared them illegal. Private adoptions are not the same thing as "black market" adoptions or baby selling. Yes, baby selling does occur, and you could come in contact with someone wanting to "give" you a baby for a hefty price. This would be unethical. No one should make a profit in adoption. With private adoption, everything is aboveboard and you'd simply be reimbursing the birth mother for certain expenses. The birth mother should not make a profit by relinquishing her baby for adoption.

At any rate, after hiring a lawyer, the next obvious step in the process would be to locate a mother who wanted to give up her child for adoption. As you may imagine, this is easier said than done. But, rest assured, there are women out there who want to give up their babies for adoption—you just have to find them.

One person who might be able to instruct you in the best methods for making such contacts could be your lawyer. If your lawyer has a lot of experience, he will have no doubt seen both successful and unsuccessful adoptions, and he should be able to tell you a little something about what will and won't work in your area. Another source, again, is an adoption support group; the members of these groups could no doubt relate some of the methods they've used to find birth mothers.

By and large, though, a prime way of locating a birth mother is simply by word of mouth. Most adoption counselors tell their clients—once they've decided to adopt—to tell everyone they know and meet about their desire to adopt a baby. The reason for this is the hope that, eventually, they'd talk with someone who knew a woman who was pregnant and thinking about adoption.

Many couples choose to augment their verbal search for a birth mother by placing advertisements in newspapers or magazines. Be forewarned, though, that advertising for a baby is illegal in 18 states. If you happen to live in one of those states, you'd need to intensify your word-of-mouth campaign. Some couples try to get around the ban on advertising by preparing elaborate résumés describing themselves and their desire for a child; they then mail these résumés to anyone who might know a pregnant woman who's considering relinquishing her child for adoption. Some possible targets include doctors; ministers, priests, or rabbis; and even school counselors. Technically, this is still advertising; even so, most states won't prohibit such efforts. But, to be on the safe side, you'd want to consult your lawyer before implementing such direct mail tactics.

To receive the responses that result from their inquiries, most couples install a separate telephone line. That way, whenever the phone rings, they know it's someone calling about their adoption request. Be prepared, though; you're bound to receive more than a few false leads and some crank calls. But if you stick with your search, you'd eventually make the contact that could change your life.

Once you'd identified a birth mother, your next step would depend, at least to some degree, on you and your desires. You may choose to maintain as much privacy as possible, in which case you'd arrange for all communication between you and the birth mother to occur through your lawyer. On the other hand, you may want to meet with the birth mother so that everyone can get to know each other. Regardless of your desires, your state government has something to say about this aspect of private adoption, too. Some states allow the adopting couple and the birth parents to remain anonymous, if they so desire; other states require the parties involved to share information about themselves with each other. The spirit of the law is that all parties become thoroughly acquainted; however, many couples try to limit the information exchanged to vital statistics, such as name, address, and age. Once again, this is where a good lawyer should be your guide.

After handling the initial contact, you'd want to formulate an agreement with the birth mother regarding the adoption and spelling out what you would and wouldn't pay. Again, state law dictates the types of expenses that an adopting couple may assume. In general, couples adopting privately agree to cover the woman's medical expenses not covered by insurance as well as her legal expenses. (The birth mother must have her own lawyer to make sure that her interests are represented fairly.) Medical expenses vary tremendously, depending upon whether the delivery is a normal vaginal delivery or a cesarean section. Another factor influencing the outlay for medical care is the infant. If the infant has problems at birth and requires special care, costs could soar. Depending upon the laws in a particular state, other expenses the adoptive parents may wish to assume include maternity clothes, housing costs, birthing classes, and even transportation to doctor's appointments. Counseling is an optional expense, but one that could be well worth the money.

As you can see, the final cost of a private adoption will vary. If you advertise, the cost of the adoption could escalate. Placing ads in several high-circulation newspapers could run you $600 to $700 each month. Legal fees would cost another $3000 to $4000. Medical expenses would be several thousand dollars more, although this would vary greatly depending on whether complications arose. As a general rule, though, a private adoption will cost somewhere between $15,000 and $20,000, although it could cost much more.

Throughout this process, you'd need to be wary about agreeing to pay any expenses that couldn't be fully documented. It's going to be up to you to make sure the adoption you're arranging doesn't turn into a black market adoption. Just remember: no one should make a profit, including the mother. You should also know that all money paid to the birth mother will be closely scrutinized by the courts, which must approve the adoption petition. A judge usually won't sanction a large, lump-sum payment to a birth mother, even if she claims to have lost her job because of the pregnancy.

A major risk in a private adoption is that the birth mother could change her mind and back out of the agreement at any step along the way. If you'd already paid some of her medical bills or advanced her money for living expenses, you'd probably never see that money again. This leads to the second risk with private adoption, and that's that you'd get involved with someone who had no intention of relinquishing her baby, but who would string you along just for the money. These things *do* happen, so beware.

If all goes well, though, the mother would give birth to a healthy infant and you'd be there to pick the baby up and bring it home. Of course, the baby wouldn't be legally yours at that point. Most states will require that you undergo a home study, which would be performed by a court representative or a social worker suggested by your lawyer. (A few states require that the home study be completed before the child is placed in the home.) The same social worker who interviewed you would also visit the birth mother. Her primary reason for doing so would be to make sure that the birth mother's story about the adoption matched yours and that she wasn't being coerced into giving up her baby.

Sometime in here the birth mother would have to sign the papers relinquishing her rights to the baby. Exactly when and how this would occur will vary according to the state in which the baby is born. Some states have a waiting period after the birth of the baby before the relinquishment can be legally signed. Other states insist that the birth mother sign the relinquishment papers in front of a judge. In still other states, a licensed adoption agency has to be involved. A few states require the birth mother to sign two sets of papers: one immediately after the birth and the other several months later. Also, in most states, the putative father must also sign documents relinquishing his rights to the baby. At any rate, you'd want to be certain that the process was followed to the letter. A fraudulently obtained consent is the primary reason that a court will nullify or void an adoption.

The bottom line in all of this, though, is that you'd have the baby for some time before the relinquishment papers were ever signed. This means that you'd run the risk of having the mother change her mind and ask for the baby back. Even after the relinquishment is signed, the birth parents could still reclaim their child for a certain period of time. Exactly how long they'd have before the courts would no longer consider such a claim varies from state to state.

These are some real risks involved with adopting privately. Some couples have supported a birth mother—both financially and emotionally—for months, only to have the birth mother change her mind at the last minute. Although the statistics for failed private adoptions are difficult to gather, the National Committee for Adoption estimates that about 20% of private adoptions fail because of legal or other problems.[5]

Although you need to be aware of the risks of private adoption, at the same time, don't forget the advantages. For starters, the waiting period is much less than with an agency adoption. If you find a birth mother quickly, you could have your baby in less than a year. Another advantage is that you'd get to bring your adopted baby home immediately after birth instead of having to wait until all of the paperwork was completed. Furthermore, with a private adoption, you wouldn't have to endure the prying of an agency. A private adoption would also give you a great deal of control. Instead of just waiting passively for something to occur, you'd be working to make things happen. And, finally, you'd have the option of getting to know the birth parents. This could be a definite plus when your child begins to wonder about his birth parents. Of course, you wouldn't be required to have a lot of contact with the birth parents if you didn't want to. Some couples aren't comfortable with such contact and prefer to deal with the birth mother only through an intermediary before the birth and then sever contact after the birth. Either way, the choice would be yours.

All in all, private adoption has its risks; but it has its advantages, too. Perhaps the biggest advantage of all is that it gives couples who might not have the chance to adopt through an agency the opportunity to become parents.

Foreign Adoption

Because of the shortage of healthy infants available for adoption in the United States, more and more families are seeking to adopt children from other parts of the world. The most common countries from which Americans adopt children include Korea, the Philippines, India, Columbia, and Chile.

As with anything else, there are advantages and disadvantages to foreign adoption. One advantage is that, because these countries tend to have more infants available than does the United States, foreign adoption agencies usually have more relaxed criteria when selecting adoptive parents. Also, you'd probably be able to adopt a child much quicker from a foreign agency than you would from an agency in the United States. However, a foreign adoption isn't any cheaper than a domestic adoption, and, because you'd have to deal with several state and national agencies, the paperwork can be even more overwhelming than it is with domestic adoptions. You'd also have to be more diligent when dealing with a foreign agency than you would if you were dealing with an agency in the United States. Keep in mind that foreign agencies don't have to follow U.S. law; therefore, there's nothing to stop them—except your diligence—from charging you an exorbitant fee or performing an adoption that's illegal.

Adopting a child from a foreign country requires that a couple do some serious soul-searching. Both you and your partner would need to seriously consider whether you'd be comfortable raising a child who was of a different race and culture. When having these discussions, you should also try to think about which cultures hold a special interest for you. You need to consider that, one day, you'd want to teach the child about his heritage. If you are truly fascinated by that foreign culture, this task will not only be more enjoyable for you, it will have much more meaning for the child.

If you decide to adopt a child from another country, you could go about this by any one of several ways. One way is to consult an adoption agency in the United States that handles these types of adoptions. Again, an agency is probably the safest way to complete a foreign adoption, but it's not your only choice. Another option is to work through a facilitator, who would serve as an intermediary between you and the adoption agency in the other country. Of course, you could work with the foreign agency yourself, but you'd need to hire a translator if you didn't speak the language. Another possibility would be to work with a lawyer in the particular country where you want to adopt a child. Of all of the methods, this is probably the riskiest. While some lawyers are completely trustworthy, others aren't. In this type of situation, it would be easy for an unethical lawyer to take your money and never follow through on an adoption.

Needless to say, the steps to completing a foreign adoption will vary depending on the method you choose and also the country involved. If you work with an agency in the United States, the process would begin just like a domestic adoption. You'd start by going to an orientation meeting at an agency and filling out an application. Then, you'd go through an interview and a home study process. The topics covered during the home study may vary, depending upon the country in question. You'd also gather the same documents that you'd gather for a domestic adoption, such as birth and marriage certificates and financial statements. But besides that, the documents going to the foreign country would have to be notarized and verified. This involves sending the notarized documents to your state's Secretary of State, who would verify the notary as legitimate. After that, the foreign country's consulate would inspect the documents before approving them as being authentic. Then, finally, the documents would have to be translated into the language of the other country.

Quite a process, to be sure, but once all of the documents

were in and you'd been approved by both the foreign and domestic agencies, you'd receive pictures and biographical sketches from the foreign agencies about the children who were available. Once you decided on a child who seemed just right for you, the U.S. agency would notify the foreign agency, who would then send that particular child's birth certificate along with proof that the child had been relinquished by the birth mother. At that point, you'd contact the U.S. Immigration and Naturalization Service (INS) to begin the extensive paperwork process of bringing your child home.

First, you'd complete a form from the INS to classify the child you wanted to adopt as an immediate relative who is an orphan. At this same time, you'd have to submit your fingerprints, proof of U.S. citizenship, your marriage certificate, and the report of your home study. Be forewarned that this is not a quick process. Just having your fingerprints checked and approved can take up to three months.

After the INS approved your petition, you'd contact the State Department to obtain a visa and a passport for the child. The U.S. consulate in that particular country would issue these documents, after which the child would be free to come to the United States. In some situations, a social worker may bring the child to you. Many foreign countries, though, require one or both prospective parents to travel to that country and stay until the paperwork is completed; this could take anywhere from two days to a month.

Once your child was finally in the United States, you'd have to register him as an alien with the INS. This would mark the beginning of your probationary period, during which a social worker would periodically check on your situation. Depending on the country involved, the probationary period would last from six months to a year. If everything goes well, once the probationary period was over, you'd go to court to finalize the adoption. The very last step would be to begin the process of having the child declared a naturalized citizen.

When considering adopting a child from a foreign country,

you need to realize that you may know little about the child's background. Most of these children were born into poverty; therefore, you'd have to assume that the child had received little or no medical care. If you work through an agency, you're likely to know more about any medical problems than you would if you were to handle the adoption privately. Many foreign children adopted by U.S. couples arrive in this country malnourished, with intestinal parasites, or without adequate immunizations. However, these deficiencies can usually be easily remedied within a short period of time. You shouldn't let these minor problems overshadow the advantage of being able to adopt a baby, first of all, and then of being able to adopt in a shorter period of time than would have been possible with a domestic agency.

Special Needs Children

When you're considering all of your adoption options, you should also consider whether you'd be willing to adopt a child who is older or who has some type of a special need. This special need could be a severe handicap, such as mental retardation, cerebral palsy, or blindness. Or, the child might only have a minor disability that could be remedied, such as a cleft palate or mild deafness.

Adopting such a child can have its own special rewards. Besides that, the adoption process is likely to move quickly, and, furthermore, some government adoption agencies pay subsidies to parents who adopt children with special needs.

If you choose to adopt such a child, the process would begin with an application and a home study, just like with any other agency adoption. But then the process would differ. Instead of waiting years to be contacted about one infant who was available, the agency would tell you about all of the adoptable children, allowing you to choose. In many instances, an agency allows the prospective parents to meet the children beforehand to help them make up their minds.

Adopting a child with special needs isn't for everyone. But give it some thought. Who knows? It could be just right for you.

Conclusion

Adoption is certainly an option if you find you can't have children of your own. But if you postpone parenthood past a certain point, you may find that even your adoption options are limited. For example, you wouldn't be able to adopt through an agency.

This chapter presented only a very brief overview of adoption to help you understand just what's involved in such a process. If you reach the point where you are truly considering adopting a child, you'll need much more information than what was presented here. Besides the fact that the laws regulating adoption change, the number of children available through agency, private, or foreign adoption changes. So, when the time is right, seek out as much information as you can, preferably through your own reading as well as through personal contacts. Adoption is an option, to be sure; it will just require diligence and effort on your part to transform the possibility of adoption into a reality.

EPILOGUE

Making the Choice

Identifying the best time to have children is never easy. But, because of the information presented in this book, you now can base your decision on more than just whim—you can base it on fact.

By this point, you know a lot about aging. You know the details of how your age affects your chances for becoming pregnant and for delivering a normal, healthy infant. You even know how your age can influence the emotional development of your child once you do give birth. But, while considering these crucial bits of information, don't overlook the fact that a few extra years of age can give your life a maturity and completeness for which there can be no substitute. It bears repeating that parents who are older are typically calmer, more financially secure, and more willing to devote their energies to raising a child than are parents who are younger. With age, it may take you longer to become a parent, but, when you do, you're likely to be a *better* parent than if you'd conceived before you were ready.

But more than knowing the facts about age and fertility, you now also know how to maintain your reproductive fitness until you wish to conceive. Throughout your years of postponement, guard your reproductive health with the same zeal that you'd guard the health of your heart or any other vital organ. Be alert for any sign of a problem and then, if one becomes apparent, seek help immediately. Even if you're not ready to conceive at that point, seeking help early could be a deciding factor in whether or not you'll be able to conceive when you're ready— even if that doesn't happen to be for several more years.

If you find that you do need expert medical attention, use the information in this book to help you select an appropriate specialist and then to guide you through the maze of diagnostic tests and infertility treatments. Always bear in mind that your reproductive health is a priceless, irreplaceable commodity. Don't mindlessly entrust that commodity to anyone—not even your doctor. If having children later in life is important to you, then you must assume the responsibility of making sure that you receive the care you need.

You have a lot to think about, to be sure. However, don't let yourself be overwhelmed by the number of things that can go wrong with the reproductive system. The point of this book is *not* to encourage you to hurry up and have children before you develop a problem with infertility. The point is simply to give you the facts you need so that you can make your own personal decision about how late to wait before trying to become pregnant.

Postponing parenthood carries with it certain risks, there's no denying it. You risk not being able to conceive quickly or without medical intervention; you even risk not being able to conceive at all. But, at the same time, postponing parenthood brings with it certain benefits—mainly the benefit of being able to focus on your own life and career before you have to devote your attention and energy to raising a child.

Unfortunately, there is no way to know in advance if your decision to delay childbearing will cause you any problem when you try to conceive. This uncertainty only makes your decision that much more difficult. But that's life—there are no guarantees. The one certainty is that, if you want to gain something, you'll probably have to give up something else. This definitely applies to parenthood. The important thing is to make your decision about when to become a parent intelligently. Analyze the risks you face by postponing childbearing and then balance those against what you're likely to gain. Eventually the two will balance out, or you may even find that you're risking more than you're gaining. When that happens, you'll know that the time is probably right for you to try to conceive. Good luck.

Preconception Questionnaire

The following questionnaire was developed by the Office of Technology Assessment to help young men and women learn if they're at risk for being infertile. Taking this quiz could teach you something about your own reproductive health.

Questions for Men

Do you feel that having children is very important to your goals in life?

If you do, you should develop 5- to 10-year life plans that will include the opportunity to conceive and have children.

Have you considered the role of children in a marriage and, if you are in a long-term relationship, reached an understanding regarding the number of children and when you plan to have them?

If you are involved in a significant relationship, you should initiate discussion on these issues.

Have you had unprotected intercourse for more than one year without your partner becoming pregnant?

You or your partner may be infertile.

True (yes) or false (no), a woman is only fertile one day a month.

If you answered no, you may misunderstand the relationship between timing of sex and pregnancy. Seek further information.

Have both of your testes been in your scrotum since birth? If not, have you had surgery or hormonal treatment?

Consult your physician.

Are you experiencing, or have you experienced, frequent urination or a discharge or burning during urination?

You may have an infection that could affect your fertility and that of women with whom you have had sex. See your physician and tell your sex partner(s) to see one also.

Is one of your testes significantly larger than the other?

You could have a low sperm count. Consult your physician.

Have you ever had a lump in the groin, or significant pain of the testes or scrotum?

You could have a varicocele or varicose vein in the scrotum. Consult your physician, who may examine your scrotum and do a semen analysis and sperm count.

Do you use alcohol, cigarettes, marijuana, cocaine, or prescription drugs?

Use of these products may reduce your fertility. Seek further information regarding their potential effects on your fertility.

Have you been exposed to radiation, chemotherapy, pesticides, or other chemicals, or to diethylstilbestrol (DES) when your mother was pregnant with you?

You could have decreased sperm production as a result of this exposure. Consult your physician, who may do a semen analysis and sperm count.

Have you ever had an operation on your testes or hernia repairs in the lower abdominal region?

You may have reduced fertility. Consult your physician.

Do you have more than 10 alcoholic drinks per week?

You may have semen abnormalities. Consult your physician, who may do a semen analysis and sperm count.

Do you frequently take hot tubs or saunas, or have other chronic heat exposure?

You may have reduced fertility.

Can you name all of your sexual partners?

Multiple sexual partners expose you to increased risk for AIDS, gonorrhea, herpes, and other conditions that can lead to infertility, significant illness, or even death. It is important to consider the consequences of your sexual activity.

Have you had difficulty in achieving or sustaining penile erections (potency) or sexual arousal (libido) sufficient to successfully initiate or complete sexual intercourse?

You could have a problem with the functioning of your testes.

Have you ever been treated for cancer or lymphoma?

You could have a low sperm count. Consult your physician.

Following urination, do you continue to dribble a few drops of urine or stain your underwear with urine?

This might affect your general health or your potential fertility. You probably have an infection of the prostate gland. Consult with your physician, who will need to examine you and possibly prescribe antibiotics.

Do you know how to avoid getting a venereal disease?

Venereal disease can be minimized by limiting the number of sexual partners and by using barrier methods of contraception (i.e., condom, diaphragm, or contraceptive sponge, in concert with foams or jellies).

Questions for Women

Do you feel that having children is very important to your goals in life?

If you do, you should develop 5- to 10-year life plans that will include the opportunity to conceive and have children.

Have you considered the role of children in a marriage and, if you are in a long-term relationship, reached an understanding regarding the number of children and when you plan to have them?

If you are involved in a significant relationship, you should initiate discussion on these issues.

Have you had unprotected intercourse for more than one year without becoming pregnant?

You or your partner may be infertile.

True (yes) or false (no), a woman is only fertile one day a month.

If you answered no, you may misunderstand the relationship between timing of sex and pregnancy. Seek further information.

Have you had a ruptured appendix and an appendectomy?

You may have pelvic adhesions reducing your fertility. Consult your physician.

Have you ever had profuse vaginal discharge associated with pelvic pain?

You may have a pelvic infection. Consult your physician to evaluate this history of infection.

Have you been exposed to radiation, chemotherapy, pesticides, or other chemicals, or to diethylstilbestrol (DES) when your mother was pregnant with you?

You may have an increased risk of pregnancy complications. Consult your physician for evaluation of DES exposure.

Is your weight significantly above or below what it should be?

Your fertility may be compromised. Seek information regarding a program for weight management.

Do you have significant amount of pain with your periods or at the time of intercourse?

You may have endometriosis, a condition associated with infertility. Consult your physician.

Have you ever been treated for fallopian tube infection, fallopian tube inflammation (salpingitis), uterine infection, or pelvic inflammatory disease?

Fallopian tube infection can cause blocked or damaged fallopian tubes that prevent pregnancy.

Are you currently using an intrauterine device (IUD) for contraception?

You are at increased risk of tubal infection, which can cause infertility. If you are using the Dalkon shield, have it removed. If you are using another type of IUD, consult your physician.

Have you noticed any increase in the amount of thickness of hair on your face, chest, or abdomen?

You could have a common hormone imbalance that might affect your general health or your potential fertility. Consult your physician who might perform laboratory testing to identify a particular abnormality.

Have you ever had an episode of abdominal pain, abnormal vaginal discharge, fever, or bleeding within a few weeks of an abortion or delivery?

You may have had a fallopian tube infection.

Do you have a white or milky discharge from your nipples that can be increased with gentle pressure?

You may have an elevated prolactin level. Consult your physician for a simple blood test.

Can you name all of your sexual partners?

Multiple sexual partners expose you to increased risk for AIDS, gonorrhea, herpes, and other conditions that can lead to infertility, significant illness, or even death. It is important to consider the consequences of your sexual activity.

Do you exercise vigorously (e.g., swimming, running, bicycling) for more than 60 minutes daily?

You may be at risk for an ovulatory problem. If you menstruate less frequently than once every 40 days, consult your physician.

Has a sexual partner ever complained of burning during urination or pain at the time of ejaculation?

Your partner may have had a sexually transmitted disease he could pass to you. Consult your physician regarding evaluation for history of infection.

Do you smoke more than one pack of cigarettes per day?

Smoking may be associated with difficulty conceiving and carrying a successful pregnancy to term. Stop smoking.

Have you ever had a pregnancy in the fallopian tube (an ectopic pregnancy)?

You may have fallopian tube damage.

Are you considering postponing childbearing beyond age 30 for work, school, or personal reasons?

Fertility decreases with age. You might wish to have children sooner.

Did you have your first menstrual period at the same time as your classmates?

If you had a delay of several years in the time of your first menstrual period, you are at risk for having problems with ovulation.

Do your mother or sisters have endometriosis?

You also may have endometriosis, a condition associated with infertility. Consult your physician regarding evaluation for endometriosis and a discussion of future plans for pregnancy.

Did you begin intercourse before the age of 20, have greater than five previous sexual partners, or a sexual partner with a genital infection or discharge?

Some sexually transmitted infections can produce fallopian tube damage.

Have you had any operations on your cervix, such as cone biopsy, cervical freezing, or electrocautery?

Your cervical mucus quality may be poor, which may compromise your ability to get pregnant. Consult your physician for evaluation of your cervical mucus.

Have you ever had sexual relations with a man who you think might have been homosexual, bisexual, or a drug user?

You are at increased risk for AIDS. Consult your physician to decide whether you should have a test for AIDS.

Did your mother experience menopause before the age of 40?

You could also experience early menopause. Consult your physician.

Have you had two or more voluntary abortions?

Use effective birth control to prevent cervical injury, uterine scarring, or pelvic infection from repeated abortions.

Do your menstrual periods last longer than 6 days, come more frequently than every 24 days, or require the use of both a tampon and pad together to maintain cleanliness during your period?

These factors are associated with a lack of regular ovulation.

Do you know how to avoid getting a venereal disease?

Venereal disease can be minimized by limiting the number of sexual partners and by using barrier methods of contraception (i.e., condom, diaphragm, or contraceptive sponge, in concert with foams or jellies).

Of the following, which do you think may affect your fertility: weight loss, weight gain, dieting, exercise, hormone pills, or stress?

All these factors can prevent regular ovulation.

APPENDIX B

Resources

If you'd like more information about any of the topics covered in this book, the following groups are a good place to start. This is, by no means, an inclusive list of the resources or support groups available. But, besides being able to provide you with some valuable information, many of these groups could also point you toward other groups if you find you need more specialized information.

Resolve, Inc.
1310 Broadway
Somerville, MA 02144-1731
(617) 623-0744

National support group for infertile couples with local chapters throughout the United States. They maintain a referral list of infertility specialists, have an extensive lending library and list of publications for sale, and also have an R.N. on staff to answer questions regarding infertility treatments. Besides dealing with infertility issues, Resolve is a great resource for adoption information, and they are also active in trying to enact legislation regarding insurance coverage for infertility treatments.

American Fertility Society
2140 Eleventh Avenue South
Suite 200
Birmingham, AL 35205-2800

A society that provides regional lists of physician members but makes no recommendations. Besides maintaining a thorough recommended reading list, the society has also produced a book detailing the success various clinics have had with assisted reproductive technologies (such as IVF, GIFT, and ZIFT).

March of Dimes Birth Defects Foundation
1275 Mamaroneck Avenue
White Plains, NY 10605

A voluntary organization that provides information on prenatal care, prevention of birth defects, and infant mortality. Contact your local chapter for specific information.

Planned Parenthood Federation of America
810 Seventh Avenue
New York, NY 10019

Organization that provides information on sexually transmitted diseases, contraceptive devices, and other aspects of a woman's reproductive health. They have numerous chapters in cities throughout the United States.

National Committee for Adoption
1930 17th Street N.W.
Washington, DC 20009-6207

Nonprofit organization that focuses on adoption of infants with special needs. They will provide lists of agencies that place such infants as well as agencies specializing in international adoption. They publish a newsletter and also have an extensive list of recommended publications available for purchase. Perhaps their most significant publication is *The Adoption Factbook*; besides discussing the various types of adoptions, this book also has an extensive list of resources and support groups.

Adoptive Families of America
3333 Highway 100 North
Minneapolis, MN 55422

This is a support organization for families who have already adopted; however, they will send, free of charge, a book about adoption to anyone who is thinking about adopting a child. They also publish a magazine aimed at adoptive parents, and sell books about such issues as raising adoptive children as well as books aimed at children who have been adopted.

*   *   *

Special Note: If you're interested in adopting through an agency, you should contact the government agency in your state that deals with adoption issues. To locate this agency, look in your telephone book (or ask the operator) for the state department that is designated to deal with health and social issues (such as the Department of Health and Human Services, although the name will vary with each state). This department will most likely be located in your state's capital. From there, you'll be able to locate the specific agency that handles adoption; this agency can then guide you to the agencies licensed by your state to place children with adoptive families.

References

Introduction

1. "Postponed Childbearing—United States, 1970–1987," *Journal of the American Medical Association*, 263 (January 19, 1990), p. 360.
2. Doug Podolsky, "Having Babies Past 40," *U.S. News & World Report*, 2 (October 29, 1990), p. 105.
3. Ibid.
4. Machelle M. Seibel, "Workup of the Infertile Couple," in *Infertility: A Comprehensive Text*, ed. Machelle M. Seibel (Norwalk, Connecticut: Appleton & Lange, 1990), p. 2.
5. Philip Elmer-Dewitt, "Making Babies," *Time*, 138 (September 30, 1991), p. 56.
6. Jane Menken, James Trussell, and Ulla Larsen, "Age and Infertility," *Science*, 233 (September 26, 1986), p. 1393.
7. Ibid.

Chapter 1

1. Machelle M. Seibel, "Workup of the Infertile Couple," in *Infertility: A Comprehensive Text*, ed. Machelle M. Seibel (Norwalk, Connecticut: Appleton & Lange, 1990), p. 2.
2. Ibid.

Chapter 2

1. Jane Menken, James Trussell, and Ulla Larsen, "Age and Infertility," *Science*, 233 (September 26, 1986), pp. 1389–1394.
2. G. E. Hendershot, W. D. Mosher, and W. F. Pratt, "Infertility and Age: An Unresolved Issue," *Family Planning Perspectives*, 14 (5), (1982) pp. 287–290.
3. Ibid.
4. D. Schwartz and M. J. Mayaux, "Female Fecundity as a Function of Age," *New England Journal of Medicine*, 306 (February 18, 1982), pp. 404–406.
5. John Bongaarts, "Infertility After Age 30: A False Alarm," *Family Planning Perspectives*, 14 (March/April 1982), pp. 75–78.
6. Gerry E. Hendershott, "Maternal Age and Overdue Conceptions," *American Journal of Public Health*, 74 (January 1984), pp. 35–38.
7. W. D. Mosher, "Infertility Trends Among U.S. Couples: 1965–1976," *Family Planning Perspectives*, 14 (January/February 1982), pp. 23–27.
8. Doug Podolsky, "Having Babies Past 40," *U.S. News & World Report*, 2 (October 29, 1990), p. 105.
9. William James, "The Causes of the Decline in Fecundability with Age," *Social Biology*, 26 (Winter 1979), pp. 330–334.
10. Paul R. Grindoff and Raphael Jewelewicz, "Reproductive Potential in the Older Woman," *Fertility and Sterility*, 46 (December 1986), pp. 989–1001.
11. Menken, pp. 1389–1394.
12. Machelle M. Seibel, "Workup of the Infertile Couple," in *Infertility: A Comprehensive Text*, ed. Machelle M. Seibel (Norwalk, Connecticut: Appleton & Lange, 1990), p. 6.
13. Menken, pp. 1389–1394.
14. J. Trussell and C. Wilson, *Population Studies*, 39 (1985).
15. Menken, pp. 1389–1394.
16. M. P. Vessey, N. H. Wright, K. McPherson, and P. Wiggins, "Fertility After Stopping Different Methods of Contraception," *British Medical Journal*, 1 (February 4, 1978), pp. 265–267.
17. Menken, pp. 1389–1394.
18. J. A. Collins et al., "Treatment-Independent Pregnancy Among Infertile Couples," *New England Journal of Medicine*, 309 (November 17, 1983), pp. 1201–1206.
19. Bongaarts, pp. 75–78.

Chapter 3

1. Machelle M. Seibel, "Workup of the Infertile Couple," in *Infertility: A Comprehensive Text*, ed. Machelle M. Seibel (Norwalk, Connecticut: Appleton & Lange, 1990), p. 8.
2. Jo Ann Rosenfeld, "Pregnancy in Women Over 35," *Postgraduate Medicine*, 87 (February 1, 1990), pp. 167–169, 172.
3. Joseph H. Bellina and Josleen Wilson, *You Can Have A Baby* (New York: Crown Publishers, 1985), p. 335.
4. Seibel, p. 8.
5. Ibid.
6. Doug Podolsky, "Having Babies Past 40," *U.S. News & World Report*, 2 (October 29, 1990), p. 105.
7. David Hollander and James L. Breen, "Pregnancy in the Older Gravida: How Old Is Old?" *Obstetrical and Gynecological Survey*, 45 (February 1990), pp. 106–112.
8. Podolsky, p. 105.
9. Gina Kolata, "As Fears about a Fetal Test Grow, Many Doctors Are Advising against It," *The New York Times* (July 15, 1992), p. B-7.
10. Ibid.
11. Rosenfeld, p. 168.
12. D. A. Grimes and G. K. Gross, "Pregnancy Outcomes in Black Women Aged 35 and Older," *Obstetrics and Gynecology*, 58 (November 1981), pp. 614–619.
13. Hollander, p. 111.
14. Grimes, pp. 614–619.
15. Rosenfeld, p. 168.
16. D. Kirz, W. Dorchester, and R. Freeman, "Advanced Maternal Age: The Mature Gravida," *American Journal of Obstetrics and Gynecology*, 152 (May 1, 1985), pp. 7–11.
17. Gertrude S. Berkowitz, "Delayed Childbearing and Outcome of Pregnancy," *New England Journal of Medicine*, 322 (March 8, 1990), pp. 659–664.
18. William N. Spellacy, Stephen J. Miller, and Ann Winegar, "Pregnancy After 40 Years of Age," *Obstetrics and Gynecology*, 68 (October 1986), p. 452.
19. I. Morrison, "The Elderly Primigravida," *American Journal of Obstetrics and Gynecology*, 121 (February 15, 1975), p. 465.
20. Kirz, p. 8.
21. Berkowitz, p. 659.

22. Kirz, p. 9.
23. Hollander, p. 111.
24. Kirz, p. 11.
25. Ibid.
26. Berkowitz, p. 659.
27. Robert A. Hahn and Suresh H. Moolgavkar, "Nulliparity, Decade of First Birth, and Breast Cancer in Connecticut Cohorts, 1855 to 1945: An Ecological Study," *American Journal of Public Health*, 79 (November 1989), p. 1503.
28. Kirz, p. 7.
29. Spellacy, p. 452.

Chapter 4

1. Stanley Coren, "Left-handedness in Offspring as a Function of Maternal Age at Parturition," *New England Journal of Medicine*, 322 (June 7, 1990), p. 1673.
2. I. C. McManus, "Left-handedness and Maternal Age," *New England Journal of Medicine*, 323 (November 14, 1990), pp. 1426–1428.
3. Arlene S. Ragozin, Robert B. Bashane, Keith A. Crnic, Mark T. Greenberg, and Nancy M. Robinson, "Effects of Maternal Age on Parenting Role," *Developmental Psychology*, 18 (July 1982), p. 627.
4. National Center for Health Statistics, *Advance Report of Final Natality Statistics*, 1987.
5. Ross D. Parke, "Families in a Life-Span Perspective," in *Child Development in Life-Span Perspective*, ed. E. M. Hetherington, R. M. Lerner, and M. Perlmutter (Hillsdale, New Jersey: Lawrence Erlbaum Associates, 1988), p. 181.
6. Andrew L. Yarrow, *Latecomers: Children of Parents Over 35* (New York: The Free Press, 1991), p. 163.
7. Monica Morris, *Last Chance Children: Growing Up with Older Parents* (New York: Columbia University Press, 1988), p. 136.
8. Yarrow, p. 138.
9. Morris, p. 151.
10. Yarrow, pp. 155–156.
11. Morris, p. 159.
12. Ibid.
13. Alison Clarke-Stewart, Susan Friedman, and Joanne Koch, *Child Development: A Topical Approach* (New York: Wiley, 1985), p. 85.

14. Martha Smilgis, "Older Parents: Good for Kids?" *Time*, 132 (October 10, 1988), pp. 98–99.

Chapter 5

1. Congress of United States, Office of Technical Assessment, "Prevention of Infertility," in *Infertility: Medical and Social Choices* (Washington, D.C.: U.S. Government Printing Office, 1988), pp. 85–92.
2. Joseph H. Bellina and Josleen Wilson, *You Can Have a Baby* (New York: Crown Publishers, 1985), p. 235.
3. Carlton A. Eddy, "The Fallopian Tube: Physiology and Pathology," in *Infertility: Diagnosis and Management*, ed. James Aiman (Berlin: Springer-Verlag, 1984), p. 171.
4. Richard L. Sweet and Ronald S. Gibbs, *Infectious Diseases of the Female Genital Tract* (Baltimore: Williams & Wilkins, 1985), p. 63.
5. Jane Menken and Ulla Larsen, "Fertility Rates and Aging," in *Aging, Reproduction, and the Climacteric*, ed. C. A. Paulsen and L. Mastroianni, Jr. (New York: Plenum Press, 1986), p. 165.
6. David W. Kaufman, Dennis Slone, Lynn Rosenberg, Olli S. Miettinen, and Samuel Shapiro, "Cigarette Smoking and Age at Natural Menopause," *American Journal of Public Health*, 70 (April 1980), pp. 420–421.
7. Hershel Jick, Jane Porter, and Alan S. Morrison, "Relation Between Smoking and Age of Natural Menopause," *The Lancet*, 1 (June 25, 1977), pp. 1354–1355.
8. Sakari Sunonio, et al., "Smoking Does Affect Fecundity," *European Journal of Obstetrics and Gynecology and Reproductive Biology*, 34 (January/February 1990), pp. 89–95.
9. D. D. Baird and A. J. Wilcox, "Cigarette Smoking Associated with Delayed Conception, *Journal of the American Medical Association*, 253 (May 24, 1985), p. 2979.
10. G. M. Tokutata, "Smoking in Relation to Infertility and Fetal Loss," *Archives of Environmental Health*, 17 (September 1968), p. 353.
11. Machelle M. Seibel, "Workup of the Infertile Couple," in *Infertility: A Comprehensive Text*, ed. Machelle M. Seibel (Norwalk, Connecticut: Appleton & Lange, 1990), p. 5.
12. Ibid., p. 6.
13. John R. Sussman and B. Blake Levitt, *Before You Conceive: The Complete Prepregnancy Guide* (New York: Bantam Books, 1989), pp. 22, 23.

14. Deborah Marquardt, "New Trends in Pregnancy Care," *McCall's*, 117 (January 1990), pp. 51–52.
15. Sussman, p. 28.
16. Bellina, p. 300.
17. John Queenan and Kimberly Leslie, "A Case for Preplanning," *Health*, 21 (December 1989), pp. 38–39, 86.
18. Marian Sandmaier, "The Weight Factor," *Working Woman*, 16 (January 1991), p. 97.
19. M. Riduan Joesoef, et al., "Are Caffeinated Beverages Risk Factors for Delayed Conception?" *The Lancet*, 335 (January 20, 1990), pp. 136–137.
20. Sussman, p. 233.
21. D. A. Metzger, D. L. Olive, G. R. Stohs, and R. R. Franklin, "Association of Endometriosis and Spontaneous Abortion: Effect of Control Group Selection," *Fertility and Sterility*, 45 (January 1986), pp. 18–22.
22. Robert D. Wayne, *Endometriosis*, brochure (Waverly, New York: Medfax-Sentinel, 1988).
23. Steven R. Bayer and Machelle M. Seibel, "Endometriosis: Pathophysiology and Treatment," in *Infertility: A Comprehensive Text*, ed. Machelle M. Seibel (Norwalk, Connecticut: Appleton & Lange, 1990), p. 120.
24. Ibid.
25. Ibid.
26. The American Fertility Society, "The Evaluation of Tubal and Peritoneal Factors," in *Investigation of the Infertile Couple*, p. 12, as quoted in "Consumer Protection Issues Involving In Vitro Fertilization Clinics," *Hearing before the Subcommittee on Regulation, Business Opportunities, and Energy of the Committee on Small Business*, March 9, 1989 (Washington, D.C.: U.S. Government Printing Office), p. 38.
27. Sussman, pp. 238–239.
28. Bellina, p. 265.
29. Sharon B. Jaffe and Raphael Jewelewicz, "The Basic Infertility Investigation," *Fertility and Sterility*, 56 (October 1991), p. 602.

Chapter 6

1. Gregory H. Corsan, Dolly Ghazi, and Ekkehard Kemmann, "Home Urinary Luteinizing Hormone Immunoassays: Clinical Applications," *Fertility and Sterility*, 53 (April 1990), pp. 591–601.

2. John R. Sussman and B. Blake Levitt, *Before You Conceive* (New York: Bantam Books, 1989), p. 132.
3. Michael Specter, "Intensive Exercise Reported to Impair Women's Fertility," *The Washington Post*, 113 (February 15, 1988), p. A-1.
4. Alice D. Domar, Machelle M. Seibel, and Herbert Benson, "The Mind/Body Program for Infertility: A New Behavioral Treatment Approach for Women with Infertility," *Fertility and Sterility*, 53 (February 1990), pp. 246–249.
5. *Ibid.* pp. 248–249.
6. Machelle M. Seibel, "Workup of the Infertile Couple," in *Infertility: A Comprehensive Text*, ed. Machelle M. Seibel (Norwalk, Connecticut: Appleton & Lange, 1990), p. 6.
7. R. J. Levine, R. M. Mathew, C. B. Chenault, M. H. Brown, N. E. Hurtt, K. S. Bentley, K. L. Mohr, and P. K. Working, "Differences in the Quality of Semen in Outdoor Workers During Summer and Winter," *The New England Journal of Medicine*, 323 (July 5, 1990), pp. 12–16.

Chapter 7

1. Machelle M. Seibel, "Workup of the Infertile Couple," in *Infertility: A Comprehensive Text*, ed. Machelle M. Seibel (Norwalk, Connecticut: Appleton & Lange, 1990), p. 3.
2. Ibid.
3. Carlton A. Eddy, "The Fallopian Tube: Physiology and Pathology," in *Infertility: Diagnosis and Management*, ed. James Aiman (Berlin: Springer-Verlag, 1984), p. 170.
4. Gilbert G. Haas, Jr., and Phillip C. Galle, "The Cervix in Reproduction," in *Infertility: Diagnosis and Management*, ed. James Aiman (Berlin: Springer-Verlag, 1984), p. 124.
5. Ibid., p. 8.
6. Joseph H. Bellina and Josleen Wilson, *You Can Have a Baby* (New York: Crown Publishers, 1985), p. 107.
7. Office of Technology Assessment, "OTA finds infertility a $1 billion problem," *Science News*, 133 (May 21, 1988), p. 327.
8. Ibid.

Chapter 8

1. The American Fertility Society, "Endocrine Factors in Female Infertility," in *Investigation of the Infertile Couple*, p. 8, as quoted in "Con-

sumer Protection Issues Involving In Vitro Fertilization Clinics," *Hearing before the Subcommittee on Regulation, Business Opportunities, and Energy of the Committee on Small Business*, March 9, 1989 (Washington, D.C.: U.S. Government Printing Office), p. 33.

2. Judith L. Vaitukaitis, "Anovulation and Amenorrhea," in *Infertility: A Comprehensive Text*, ed. Machelle M. Seibel (Norwalk, Connecticut: Appleton & Lange, 1990), p. 54.

3. Paul R. Gindoff and Raphael Jewelewicz, "Reproductive Potential in the Older Woman," *Fertility and Sterility*, 46 (December 1986), p. 991.

4. Gindoff, p. 992.

5. Ibid., p. 998.

6. Sharon B. Jaffe and Raphael Jewelewicz, "The Basic Infertility Investigation," *Fertility and Sterility*, 56 (October 1991), p. 604.

7. Anne Colston Wentz, "Luteal Phase Inadequacy," in *Infertility: A Comprehensive Text*, ed. Machelle M. Seibel (Norwalk, Connecticut: Appleton & Lange, 1990), p. 84.

8. Anne Colston Wentz, Liliana R. Kossoy, and Robert A. Parker, "The Impact of Luteal Phase Inadequacy in an Infertile Population," *American Journal of Obstetrics and Gynecology*, 162 (April 1990), p. 937.

9. American Fertility Society, p. 8.

10. Machelle M. Seibel, "Workup of the Infertile Couple," in *Infertility: A Comprehensive Text* (Norwalk, Connecticut: Appleton & Lange, 1990), p. 13.

11. Ibid.

12. Seibel, pp. 10–11.

13. The American Fertility Society, "Evaluation of Cervical Factor," in *Investigation of the Infertile Couple*, p. 25, as quoted in "Consumer Protection Issues Involving In Vitro Fertilization Clinics," *Hearing before the Subcommittee on Regulation, Business Opportunities, and Energy of the Committee on Small Business*, March 9, 1989 (Washington, D.C.: U.S. Government Printing Office), p. 51.

14. Gilbert G. Haas, Jr., and Phillip C. Galle, "The Cervix in Reproduction," in *Infertility: Diagnosis and Management*, ed. James Aiman (Berlin: Springer-Verlag, 1984), p. 132.

15. W. Eggert-Kruse, M. Christmann, I. Gerhard, S. Pohl, K. Klinga, and B. Runnebaum, "Circulating Antisperm Antibodies and Fertility Prognosis: A Prospective Study," *Human Reproduction*, 4 (July 1989), pp. 513–518.

16. Nancy Alexander, "Treatment for Antisperm Antibodies: Voodoo or Victory?" *Fertility and Sterility*, 53 (April 1990), pp. 602–603.

17. Ibid.
18. Ehud J. Margalloth, et al., "Intrauterine Insemination as Treatment for Antisperm Antibodies in the Female," *Fertility and Sterility*, 50 (September 1988), pp. 441–446.
19. C. G. Haas, Jr., O. J. D'Cruz, and B. Denum, "Effect of Repeated Washing on Sperm-Bound Immunoglobulin G," *Journal of Andrology*, 9 (May/June, 1988) pp. 190–196.
20. Alexander, p. 603.
21. W. S. Tjoa, M. H. Smolensky, B. P. Hoi, E. Steinberger, and K. D. Smith, "Circannual Rhythm in Human Sperm Count Revealed by Serially Independent Sampling," *Fertility and Sterility*, 33 (1982), p. 454.
22. Sherman J. Silber, *How to Get Pregnant With the New Technology* (New York: Warner Books, 1991), p. 147.
23. Ibid., p. 156.
24. Sherman J. Silber, "The Relationship of Abnormal Semen Values to Pregnancy Outcome," in *Infertility: A Comprehensive Text*, ed. Machelle M. Seibel (Norwalk, Connecticut: Appleton & Lange, 1990), p. 154.

Chapter 9

1. Eli Y. Adashi, "Ovulation Initiation: Clomiphene Citrate," *Infertility: A Comprehensive Text*, ed. Machelle M. Seibel (Norwalk, Connecticut: Appleton & Lange, 1990), p. 308.
2. Bruno Lunefeld and Eitan Lunefeld, "Ovulation Induction: HMG," in *Infertility: A Comprehensive Text*, ed. Machelle M. Seibel (Norwalk, Connecticut: Appleton & Lange, 1990), p. 319.
3. Ibid.
4. Lunefeld, p. 317.
5. Ibid.
6. Lunefeld, p. 319.
7. Lunefeld, p. 320.
8. E. Confino, et al., "Transcervical Balloon Tuboplasty," *Journal of the American Medical Association*, 264 (October 24, 1990), pp. 2079–2082.
9. Robert B. Hunt, "Technical Aspects of Tubal Surgery," in *Infertility: A Comprehensive Text*, ed. Machelle M. Seibel (Norwalk, Connecticut: Appleton & Lange, 1990), p. 412.
10. Ibid.

11. Stephen J. Winters, "Evaluation and Medical Management of Male Infertility," in *Infertility: A Comprehensive Text*, ed. Machelle M. Seibel (Norwalk, Connecticut: Appleton & Lange, 1990), p. 157.
12. Sherman J. Silber, *How to Get Pregnant With the New Technology* (New York: Warner Books, 1991), p. 133.
13. Sherman J. Silber, "The Relationship of Abnormal Semen Values to Pregnancy Outcome," in *Infertility: A Comprehensive Text*, ed. Machelle M. Seibel (Norwalk, Connecticut: Appleton & Lange, 1990), p. 151.
14. Ibid.
15. Randall A. Loy and Machelle M. Seibel, "Therapeutic Insemination," in *Infertility: A Comprehensive Text*, ed. Machelle M. Seibel (Norwalk, Connecticut: Appleton & Lange, 1990), p. 199.
16. Ibid.
17. Silber, "The Relationship of Abnormal Semen Values to Pregnancy Outcome," p. 154.
18. Loy, p. 212.
19. Michael R. Virro and Alan B. Shewchuk, "Pregnancy Outcome in 242 Conceptions After Artificial Insemination with Donor Sperm and Effects of Maternal Age on the Prognosis for Successful Pregnancy," *American Journal of Obstetrics and Gynecology*, 148 (March 1, 1984), p. 522.
20. Loy, p. 212.
21. Neri Laufer, Lawrence Grunfeld, and G. John Garrisi, "In-Vitro Fertilization," in *Infertility: A Comprehensive Text*, ed. Machelle M. Seibel (Norwalk, Connecticut: Appleton & Lange, 1990), p. 498.
22. Ibid. p. 499.
23. Silber, *How to Get Pregnant with the New Technology*, p. 269.
24. Gary B. Ellis. Testimony, *Hearing before the Subcommittee on Regulation, Business Opportunities, and Energy of the Committee on Small Business*, March 9, 1989. (Washington, D.C.: U.S. Government Printing Office).
25. K. L. Harrison, et al., "Patient Age and Success in a Human IVF Programme," *Australian and New Zealand Journal of Obstetrics and Gynecology*, 3 (August 1989), pp. 326–328.
26. C. Piette, J. de Mouzon, A. Bachelot, and A. Spira, "In-Vitro Fertilization: Influence of Women's Age on Pregnancy Rates," *Human Reproduction*, 5 (January 1990), pp. 56–59.
27. Harrison, pp. 326–328.
28. Piette, p. 58.

29. Shimon Segal and Robert F. Casper, "The Response to Ovarian Hyperstimulation and In-Vitro Fertilization in Women Older than 35 Years," *Human Reproduction*, 5 (April 1990), pp. 255–257.
30. Harrison, pp. 326–328.
31. Piette, p. 59.
32. Segal, p. 257.
33. Laufer, p. 503.
34. Alexander M. Dlugi, "Gamete Intrafallopian Transfer," in *Infertility: A Comprehensive Text*, ed. Machelle M. Seibel (Norwalk, Connecticut: Appleton & Lange, 1990), p. 477.
35. David S. Guzick, Jose P. Balmaceda, Terri Ord, and Ricardo H. Asch, "The Importance of Egg and Sperm Factors in Predicting the Likelihood of Pregnancy from Gamete Intrafallopian Transfer," *Fertility and Sterility*, 52 (November 1989), pp. 795–800.
36. Ricardo H. Asch, *GIFT: Gamete Intra-Fallopian Transfer*, booklet (Norwell, Massachusetts: Serono Symposia, USA, 1990), p. 11.
37. I. Craft, et al., "Analysis of 1071 GIFT Procedures—The Case for a Flexible Approach to Treatment," *The Lancet*, 1 (May 14, 1988), pp. 1094–1097.
38. I. Craft, "Factors Affecting the Outcome of Assisted Conception," *British Medical Bulletin*, 46 (July 1990), pp. 769–782.
39. Guzick, p. 797.
40. V. A. Hulme, J. P. van der Merwe, and T. F. Kruger, "Gamete Intrafallopian Transfer as Treatment for Infertility Associated with Endometriosis," *Fertility and Sterility*, 53 (June 1990), pp. 1095–1096.
41. Mark V. Sauer, Richard J. Paulson, and Rogerio A. Lobo, "A Preliminary Report on Oocyte Donation Extending Reproductive Potential to Women Over 40," *New England Journal of Medicine*, 323 (October 25, 1990), pp. 1157–1160.
42. Hossam I. Abdalla, Rodney Baber, Angela Kirkland, Terence Leonard, Mary Power, and John W. W. Studd, "A Report on 100 Cycles of Oocyte Donation; Factors Affecting Outcome," *Human Reproduction*, 5 (November 1990), pp. 1018–1022.

Chapter 10

1. Gayle D. Rundberg, *How to Get Babies Through Private Adoption* (Bend, Oregon: Maverick Publications, 1988), p. 2.

2. Lincoln Caplan, *An Open Adoption* (New York: Farrar, Straus, & Giroux, 1990), p. 121.
3. Alice D. Domar and Machelle M. Seibel, "Emotional Aspects of Infertility," in *Infertility: A Comprehensive Text*, ed. Machelle M. Seibel (Norwalk, Connecticut: Appleton & Lange, 1990), p. 31.
4. Caplan, p. 111.
5. National Committee for Adoption, *Adoption Factbook: United States Data, Issues, Regulations and Resources* (Washington, D.C.: National Committee for Adoption, 1989), p. 172.

Index